Confessions of a Zen Narcissist

Struggles with the Illusion of Self

Larry White

ISBN: 978-1-7342989-0-1 (paperback)
ISBN: 978-1-7342989-1-8 (e-book)

Library of Congress Control Number: 2019919015

Design and production by Joanne Shwed, Backspace Ink (www.backspaceink.com)

To contact Larry White: larry@healthcarejobs.net or 318.613.8929

To Christina with love and deep appreciation

It is not easy to find happiness in ourselves,
and it is not possible to find it elsewhere.
—Anaïs Nin

Contents

Foreword by Richard Collins

I n his *Journals*, Ralph Waldo Emerson envisioned the future of literature to lie, in part, in the promise of "diaries or autobiographies—captivating books, if only a man knew how to choose among what he calls his experience that which is really his experience, and how to record truth truly."

Confessions of a Zen Narcissist is one of those captivating books. Larry White's subject is not just his experience but *that which is really his experience*. For anyone with a personality disorder, distinguishing between what they *perceive* to be their experience and that which is *really* their experience is a daily struggle, if indeed they can recognize the difference at all.

Narcissistic personality disorder (NPD) is said to be particularly impenetrable and intransigent in this way, so that to record "truth truly" should be almost impossible for someone with this disorder, as though they stood on one side of a barrier with no entry, a gateless gate.

Yet Larry White has managed to arrive at the gateless gate of his NPD with the help of two paths to telling the truth truly: psychotherapy and Zen practice. One might say that therapy brought him to the gate; meditation helped him to penetrate it. This book is the story of his journey on this parallel path on the way to realizing that which was really his experience.

Confessions of a Zen Narcissist is an admission that perhaps only a *Zen* narcissist could make. Larry White is a graduate of Deep Springs College, where he encountered Alan Watts, and Pomona College, where one of his creative writing classmates was Kris Kristofferson. He also did graduate work at Boston University. But his real education has been life itself, with all of the halting progress and heartbreaking setbacks that might assail someone with his personality disorder, and as his life unfolded along several spiritual paths.

A restless seeker his entire life, Larry has been involved in a number of fringe movements, hippie communes, drug treatment centers (running them, not entering them), and Zen communities from Pasadena to Boston and from Florida to New Mexico. He has studied with various spiritual teachers, including Yasutani Roshi,[1] Fukushima Roshi, Eido Tai Shimano Roshi, Bhagwan Shree Rajneesh (Osho), and Ken Keyes, Jr. He has undergone psychotherapy with Sheldon Kopp and several other therapists.

Larry's confessions take us from his pampered childhood with parents who encouraged him to think of himself as almost divinely "special," to his young adulthood seeking acceptance and admiration from his peers, whether as a seaman or a CEO, and through marriages to a woman who could not recognize his disorder and finally to one who could.

The connecting thread of this story—*that which is really his experience*—is found in the Preface [see "The Disorder Defined" on page 12], each point of which Larry has embodied at some point in his life—sometimes all of them sounding at once, like a cacophonic orchestra of self-doubt, self-aggrandizement, success, and failure. Yet he also realizes all the while, thanks to his spiritual quest, that there might be a way out of the string of dismal failures, both professional and personal, that constitutes his resume and has resulted from his disorder.

That way is the way of Zen: specifically, the Zen doctrine of no-self. This is the true self-doubt, doubt that the "self" actually exists in the way that the narcissist never questions. The journey is not easy. It is, however, captivating. Making the journey with Larry, we come to sympathize with the unsympathetic portrait he draws of himself, leading us to a greater understanding, perhaps, of the many people around us who suffer, more or less, from a similar distortion of their true self, the true self being, as Kōdō Sawaki said, "precisely that self I haven't thought up." Some of those people may even be—to some degree—ourselves.

—Richard Collins
Abbot, New Orleans Zen Temple

---

[1] A "Roshi" is a Zen Master.

From Narcissistic Personality Disorder to Zen

The Saga Begins

This is my journey. Perhaps my quest can bring some guidance to others who suffer from NPD. Fortunately, I had a chink in my narcissistic armor, namely my lack of success as a person and as a professional. Only this characteristic allowed me to accept my disorder when I was faced with the truth; however, many years of Zen practice helped me understand a Zen experience that apparently solved my problem with NPD. While my Zen experience resolved my NPD problem, it opened me to the awareness that truly began my Zen practice 50+ years after I began calling myself a Zen Buddhist.

This story is more than a discussion of NPD. As an exaggerated manifestation of a component of other personality disorders and of the distress of all people, NPD is a disorder centering on more than the illusion of a separate and permanent self. This illusion is common to all human beings. Our sense of self is important for our growth into adulthood, but eventually we may experience that there is no separate entity called "self." To drop the illusion of separateness is to become more completely human.

NPD seems to involve an aberrant self-consciousness that prevents one from being aware of the feelings of others. Through this distorted lens, the NPD sufferer's "reality" is viewed. While this distortion of reality is easily apparent in the person with NPD, similar distortions exist in other disorders that ultimately present with complete ignorance of other people's feelings. In "normally" functioning people, since they are self-consciously aware of others' feelings, the insight that the self is empty may be more easily seen.

It is particularly ironic—or perhaps logical—that I have spent so much of my spiritual, intellectual, and emotional energy on my practice of Zen Buddhism. Even though I had practiced for most of my life, I never experienced any Zen understanding until I was able to break out of the opaque shroud of NPD. This book is an attempt to chronicle that contradiction and that insight.

For those with NPD, it is my hope that this book will help them find a path to peace if their awareness can at least tolerate an intellectual understanding of Zen practice. For those who have a personal or professional relationship with a person with NPD, perhaps this book can help these people to be more understanding of a condition that is virtually untreatable.

I offer this book to all those suffering from NPD, and to their caregivers, as possibly providing a modicum of hope.

Narcissism, in some degree, is common to all people. Narcissistic *personality disorder*, however, is a different thing. Even the successful person with NPD—and there are many—could function much better and be happier without it. NPD is like color blindness. You can't see or emotionally understand empathy, compassion, love, or any of the nine characteristics of the disorder any more than a colorblind person can comprehend "red." The person with NPD lives in a different world where the disorder defines reality, and only this reality is intelligible. This situation is important to keep in mind as we examine my NPD and NPD in general.

The Disorder Defined

The definition of NPD is not difficult to understand. According to the *Diagnostic and Statistical Manual of Mental Disorders*, Fifth Edition[2] (or, as it is called in the helping professions, DSM), a person who manifests five or more of the following characteristics of narcissistic personality has a disorder if they:

---

[2] *Diagnostic and Statistical Manual of Mental Disorders*, Fifth Edition (Washington, DC: American Psychiatric Publishing, 2013).

1) Have a grandiose sense of self-importance (e.g., exaggerate achievements and talents and expect to be recognized as superior without commensurate achievements)

2) Are preoccupied with fantasies of unlimited success, power, brilliance, beauty, or ideal love

3) Believe that they are "special" and unique and can only be understood by, or should associate with, other special or high-status people or institutions

4) Require excessive admiration

5) Have a sense of entitlement (i.e., unreasonable expectations of especially favorable treatment or automatic compliance with their expectations)

6) Are interpersonally exploitative (i.e., take advantage of others to achieve their own end)

7) Lack empathy and are unwilling to recognize or identify with the needs of others

8) Are often envious of others or believe that others are envious of them

9) Show arrogant, haughty behaviors or attitudes

Without exaggerating, I manifested all nine characteristics—some more strongly than others. I will reference each of the characteristics parenthetically by number in the following accounts (e.g., NPD #1).

My First Zen Group

In 1965, my first wife Willo and I lived with our two children Alexandra and Geoffrey in Washington, DC. I discovered a Zen group in the area whose members were disciples of the Japanese Master Hakuun Yasutani. Interested in Zen since college, I saw myself as a serious Zen student. I had warned Willo when we were married in 1962 that my most compelling personal motivation was my Zen practice; however, it would be decades before I even caught a glimpse of Zen experience. I didn't know I had a personality disorder at that time, but I knew I was searching for something. I was also convinced that I would find it.

Willo and I signed up for a seven-day retreat with Yasutani Roshi, held in a college dorm in Maryland that was closed for summer vacation. Each of the 30 attendees had a private room. The schedule was demanding. We sat in meditation side by side for two 40-minute sessions, and during work periods we picked up stones in a sod farm next door. We ate and we slept. We had one meditation before breakfast, two more before lunch, two after lunch, and one after dinner. Twice a day we met one on one with Yasutani Roshi and his Japanese translator and chief monk, who later became Eido Tai Shimano Roshi. The meetings with Yasutani were very brief. We walked into his room, bowed three times, and sat on a cushion in front of him.

We were all working on the same koan[3]—the beginner's Mu[4]: "Does a dog have Buddha nature?"

He would ask, "What is Mu?"

If we started to speak, he rang his bell, and the meeting was over. The question had no verbal answer. I knew from my reading that demonstrating the answer required a breakthrough in awareness. As a manifestation of my NPD, I placed the whole koan process with Yasutani Roshi on a pedestal of misunderstanding. I assumed that, if my very special I "solved" Mu, I would be enlightened (whatever that meant).

During one of the rest periods, I was walking in the garden, looking at the trees and thinking about the retreat. I had the strong feeling that I was afraid of becoming enlightened because I thought I might be disappointed. I clearly didn't get it. For the next 50 years, I struggled to understand Zen and to cope with my unknown personality disorder, experiencing virtually no success with either. Zen cannot be understood, but I finally dropped the disorder.

---

[3] A "koan" is a paradoxical anecdote or riddle.

[4] "Mu" is a traditional koan.

The Genesis of My Disorder

NPD is rooted in personality dysfunctions in the family, although it may well have a biological propensity. It is inadvertently caught and not invented by the person who has it. It is family generated (or at least triggered).

Long before NPD was accepted as a personality disorder by the psychological/psychiatric communities, the Pulitzer Prize-winning novelist Booth Tarkington created a "hero" who manifested all the characteristics of the disorder. His compelling novel, *The Magnificent Ambersons*,[5] was made into a critically acclaimed movie by Orson Welles in 1942. Realistically, Tarkington brings his hero to personal and emotional defeat (or, as it is called in the novel, his "comeuppance") before he can emerge from the disorder to live a useful existence.

My family dysfunctions were apparent from the beginning. I am told that my delivery into this world in Pasadena, California, in 1935 was difficult; my mother and I nearly died. She was born over the hill in Hollywood to an upper-middle-class family with a strong, opinionated mother and a quiet, saintly father who was also deeply opinionated; both were conservative, fundamentalist Methodists. Grandmother's family had come to California in a covered wagon on the Oregon Trail. Grandfather's family raised horses in Nevada and herded them to Los Angeles for sale before he created a successful leather goods company in Los Angeles.

---

[5] Booth Tarkington, *The Magnificent Ambersons* (New York: Doubleday, Page and Co., 1918).

My father came from a farming community in rural New York, south of Watertown, which was a hundred years culturally behind the Hollywood of his future wife's family. My paternal grandfather, a wallpaper hanger and painter by trade, was a weak man, not a strong male model for my father. As Seventh Day Baptists, the family was neither devout nor fundamentalist. No two families had less in common.

My parents met at a weekly meeting of the Epworth League in the South Pasadena Methodist Church. My mother, a graduate of Occidental College, taught elementary school in Montebello. My father was still an undergraduate at the University of Southern California. He had left New York and come West four years after he graduated from high school to live with an aunt in California and to get as far away from his roots as possible. Sadly, that result is never possible. We always take our roots—and their fruits—with us.

After a four-year engagement, my parents married and bought a new house in San Gabriel in the late '30s when I was four and my sister Suzy was two. My earliest consistent memories are from our time in San Gabriel. Mother did not work but was active with women's groups, including the First Methodist Church of Pasadena and the local PTA of which she became president. Pop had a number of jobs such as a UPS driver and a door-to-door lamp and electrical appliances salesman for General Electric.

One of my earliest memories, in the first or second grade, is being told that I was "special." It's hard to remember the exact words, but I was led to believe that I was somehow exceptional. My parents continued this absurd characterization well into my 20s. When I was seeing a therapist as a young man and engaged my parents in discussions of my childhood, they informed me that the sexual intercourse that caused my conception was "unusual" and, as a result, I was a unique and special being. They even told my first wife Willo that I was "the second coming."

It sounds silly when I write these words. I am convinced that growing up with the expectation that I was destined for great things was either the genesis or at least the trigger for my NPD. I was never shown *how* to be special or *how* to do great things; it was merely taken for granted that I would excel in the nonprofit world of "good works" (NPD #3). Unlike Suzy, who never suffered from a personality disorder, I was given a grandiose sense of self-importance throughout my teenage years and was taught to expect recognition of being superior without commensurate achievements (NPD #1).

My mother was a strong pacifist and raised me to be the same. She taught me to "turn the other cheek" when I got into disagreements. My parents were protective but never taught me how to take care of myself. This culture of being the good little pacifist child of a strong and opinionated mother was another NPD trigger (NPD #5). I was simply expected to grow up and save the world.

In addition to the crazy expectations of greatness with no direction, training, or support, a major cause of my NPD was the combination of my father's weakness and my mother's strength (NPD #1 and #2). My father failed in his role of aiding me in escaping from the influence of my mother; the fact that he was also dominated by her is a good reason why this occurred.

My father, Lawrence Herman White, was called Larry. I was named Lawrence Morgan White. From birth through graduation from Pomona College, I was called Lawrie. When I went to Naval Officer Candidate School in 1959, I changed my name to Larry. The name Lawrie was significant in my life. It didn't seem masculine; it indicated that I was my mother's son and student more than my father's. My father, for example, never played sports with me or took me to sporting events. Mother tried to play the role of both father and mother with limited success. This meant that I had no male leadership or example at home, and I was not permitted to find it elsewhere.

When I was eight or nine, during the war, one of our neighbors was a prosperous probate judge who lived in a big house. He was critical of my father because he never took me to a ball game. The judge took me and his son Buddy to a professional baseball game in Detroit. I don't remember the game, but I remember the stadium and the hot dogs. I also remember Buddy's father: short, chubby, friendly, and caring enough to take his son to a ball game.

After Pearl Harbor, we became acutely aware of the war. Over our house, the night sky was frequently filled with searchlights, sometimes illuminating what we thought were enemy aircraft. An oil refinery north of us near Santa Barbara was shelled by a Japanese submarine that surfaced off the coast. Our Japanese neighbors were moved to internment camps.

The war was constantly discussed, and the news was full of terrifying stories. I thought the whole drama was a lot of fun, but Pop was scared. He was, in general, insecure and frightened by life. He was offered a good job at the Jet Propulsion Laboratory (JPL) in Pasadena, which had just opened, but he was afraid that JPL might blow up from the manufacture of explosives. Pop's employment there would have had a huge stabilizing effect on the family; instead, Pop's fear uprooted us and moved us to Royal Oak, Michigan, near Detroit.

My mother (Margaret Morgan White) didn't want to leave her parents (Thomas and Susan Morgan) with whom she was extremely close. She felt that, if she left, she would never see them again. Nevertheless, even though her parents were still alive after the war, she didn't want to return to California.

By the end of the war, we were well established in Michigan. Mother had always wanted three children, and my brother Don was born in 1945. We owned a house and had no debts. We bought a new Chevrolet as soon as the first ones rolled off the assembly line in 1946. We went ice skating in winter, and Pop took me fishing in summer. He took me to his office in Detroit and let me watch newsreels all day at a nearby theater that showed them exclusively and for free.

Living in Royal Oak was a good period for me, but Pop was sure that the Depression would resume after the war. He wanted to return to California. We sold everything except the new Chevrolet and drove back to California in 1946. The move was a disaster. There was little money during those years, and we changed neighborhoods twice. My mother went back to work as a teacher to support the family. Pop poked around at several jobs, including sales and low-level business positions.

For a time, my father sold a complicated form of life insurance an acquaintance had developed. He was good at this job, and it was highly remunerative. However, when a friend to whom he had sold the product became angry with him about the policy, he grew concerned that it might be illegal and dropped out of the business. In fact, Pop never found a stable job until he became a schoolteacher like my mother in the late 1950s, after all of us kids had left home to go to college.

Always an outspoken Republican, Pop learned that I voted for John F. Kennedy in 1960 and wrote to me, "It hurts when your own son joins the ranks of the great unwashed and votes for the something-for-nothing boys."

My father maintained his illusion of being an upstanding Republican businessman until his potential influence as a provider and a strong father figure was no longer relevant. However, when Pop was surrounded by super-liberal fellow public schoolteachers, he became an anti-Ronald Reagan liberal Democrat. Never interested in sports while I was growing up, he even became a baseball fan when the Dodgers moved to Los Angeles. My parents always achieved through affiliation.

I had a habit of saying things that hurt people or made them angry. Sometimes I did it for fun, and I enjoyed making people uncomfortable; other times, I just didn't understand how they felt. One of my elementary school-teachers in San Gabriel had a husband in the military overseas. I said something that brought back her sadness about his absence and the danger he faced, but I didn't care. Later, in Michigan, my friend Buddy and I were putting together a school presentation with some other kids. The presentation called for a leader to stand behind a podium and make a speech. I told Buddy's mother, who was directing the project, that Buddy was too short for the podium, so I should have that role.

"You are so rude," she said, "and cruel."

Such instances of a lack of empathy and a sense of entitlement were not unusual for me (NPD #5 and #7).

After we returned to California from Michigan, things got worse for me. We bought a house in Altadena. I didn't have any local friends, but I was active in the Methodist Youth Fellowship (MYF). At their summer camp, I was elected president, even though I was one of the youngest campers and only in the sixth grade. On return from camp, I had a grand mal seizure. I was told that I had had one in my sleep when I was seven and a later seizure in my sleep the night before I took a date to my first formal dance. I had three more seizures before high school: two at meals with my family just after the blessing and one in school following the flag salute.

A thorough examination determined that I had a brain dysrhythmia. All of my seizures were of the classic "grand mal" type (now called "major") in which I was fully unconscious for the full duration of the seizure. I was given prescriptions for phenobarbital and Dilantin, which I took fairly regularly until I became a Navy Reserve officer on active duty. When I was sent to cryptology school in Newport, Rhode Island, I told the navy about the drugs I was taking. An EEG determined that I no longer had a dysrhythmia. I discontinued the medication and had no additional seizures. I am convinced that the dysrhythmia was psychogenic and caused by tensions in my family life.

From the late 1940s until the early 1970s, I had a series of stress-induced physical disturbances. From my earliest memories and through the majority of my life, I had a feeling of not belonging to any reality I was experiencing. I always had a feeling of temporariness and impending doom. These physical problems increased my sense of having a tentative hold on reality. After the seizure episodes, the next manifestation of internal conflict was a series of appendicitis attacks. I never had my appendix removed because the symptoms always went away in a few hours. When the appendicitis symptoms stopped, I had frequent debilitating migraine attacks for a number of years and then a series of pyloric spasm attacks for several more years.

The grand mal seizures caused years of concern that I might have another one and precipitated a number of false auras[6] during my years at Monrovia High School in Monrovia, California. My adolescence was colored by the drama of seizures. I had a continuing and frightening memory of feeling the preseizure aura and loss of consciousness. Whenever I was in a tense psychological situation or a potentially dangerous physical situation, I felt panic about the possibility of another seizure.

I can still sense that feeling as I write more than 60 years after the last episode. The seizures seemed to have a pattern. Except for the first, which was in my sleep at age seven, all the others seemed to be brought on by tension (my first formal dance) or by ceremony (a meal-time blessing or a flag salute). I developed a reluctance to travel or be away from home, which I still feel. I felt more vulnerable to a seizure when I was in strange surroundings.

My fear of seizures and my parents' desire to protect me intensified the problem. After finishing sixth grade in Altadena, I expected to start seventh grade at Marshall Junior High. A bully in my class named Bucky threatened to harass me at the new school. I was slated to be stuffed into a trash can and

---

[6] "Auras" are feelings over your entire body prior to a seizure or convulsion that consciousness is slipping away.

rolled down a ramp in the playground. I was terrified. My parents took an action that was both loving and destructive. They arranged for me to be bused to a school in a different district in Pasadena. Trying to do what was best for me, they only amplified my frailty and my fears. Pop put notes in my lunch bag to encourage me not to be afraid of a seizure. He would have done better to teach me how to defend myself and confront my fears.

Highlighting my specialness and my sense of entitlement, my parents created and then reinforced my NPD, if only unintentionally, by trying to do what was best for me (NPD #3 and #5). They seemed to assume that there was something wrong with me that was a part of my "specialness." I don't think they ever gave up the notion that all of my NPD manifestations were related to the brain dysrhythmia that caused the seizures. Of course, they didn't know about NPD, but they were very aware of its manifestations. I doubt that they ever believed it when the navy determined that I had no brain dysrhythmia after I became a naval officer and copped to my history and my medication.

High school was not a pleasant time; I never look back on it with any fondness. It was just an unfortunate four years that I had to endure to get on with life. I was a decent student with a B+ average, but I never worked hard or applied myself. I was elected to some student government offices, but I never enjoyed what I was doing. Running for student offices was a way for me to achieve the special attention to which I felt entitled (NPD #5). Most of my free time was taken up by MYF activities. I followed the teachings of Mahatma Gandhi and considered myself a pacifist. I was happiest defending pacifism in front of a classroom of my peers. I was never a part of the most popular social group, though I wanted to be.

I'm sure that pacifism was important to me because my mother had been drilling this philosophy into my head for as long as I can remember. It had some serious negative outcomes. My mother's strong pacifism and domi-nant role in the family encouraged me not to learn to defend myself. Had I learned to box or use other martial arts, my social life with other boys would have been considerably different. I would have been "one of them," a person to be taken seriously, and I think that I would have felt better about myself. Following the life and teachings of Gandhi was just a logical step to make since pacifism was an important part of my life in high school.

One of my mother's friends had a horse that I rode several times a week. I was getting the money together to buy it when my mother told her friend to sell it to someone else. In Mother's view, I should have been spending my time in social activities. The loss of "my" horse affected me deeply, but I never discussed it or acknowledged the hurt to myself.

Mother had an image of who I was—or should be—that usually conflicted with how I saw myself. I never confronted Mother directly because she fueled my specialness and my grandiosity. She laughed when I joked that I would write a book entitled, *How I became humble,* with 25 full-page illustrations of me. (Perhaps this is that book without the pictures!) I resented Mother, and I feared her, but I enjoyed her seeing me as special and validating my NPD. Although I could not have stated it in those terms at that time, she always treated me like a platonic lover (NPD #1 and #3).

In ways big and small, Mother tried to control my every activity. She always seemed to know what I should or should not do; however, she would never be straightforward and open about her feelings. I was expected to intuit what she wanted or needed. If I didn't volunteer to do the dishes, I felt her unspoken disapproval, but she would never ask. I closed myself off from feelings and nonverbal communication to protect myself from her. (After my divorce in 1973, when my daughter Alexandra and son Geoffrey were eight and six, respectively, they spent most of 10 summers with their grandparents. Today, Alex says that she is good at reading people nonverbally because of her summer experiences with Mother.)

In ways both subtle and overt, the family seemed critical of me. This affected me deeply because I remember it as though it were yesterday. During one high-school summer vacation, I got a job as a salesman at a nursery in Monrovia. At the nursery, I was taught to prune the roots of bare root roses for customers. When I related this training to my parents and Suzy, they launched into gales of laughter when thinking of me as a gardener. They were totally dismissive that I could know anything about roses. The parenting I received seems to have been all criticism and high expectations for the future with little support in the present. I was taught to be special and entitled but was never rewarded for achievement. I was always expected to do better.

Another high school summer vacation experience is illustrative of the disorder. Through his friendship with one of the Los Angeles County supervisors, Pop got me a job in the highway department warehouse in Long Beach. I put stuff on shelves, filled orders, and did various low-level jobs.

One afternoon, an issue arose about something that was supposed to be on one of the shelves but wasn't. The boss of the facility—a short, one-armed guy who was quick to anger—and one of his senior people were standing in front of the shelf, discussing the problem. I walked up and entered the conversation. The boss grabbed me by the neck with his one arm, pushed me away, and told me to get lost.

The workers never liked the boss, so they urged me to stand up for myself and tell the district supervisor about my getting manhandled when he came on one of his frequent visits. I liked the idea of getting justice. The district supervisor suspended my boss for over a month. I was a hero.

The whole event was a setup to get back at our boss and to ridicule me because I had gotten my job through my father's connections with a county supervisor. I was easily made the butt of practical jokes because I felt important, but I was vulnerable and unaware. I had the opposite of street smarts. I just bumbled along, feeling special and missing out on what was going on around me.

It turned out all right though. The next summer, I went back to see the one-armed boss who had pushed me. He greeted me heartily, patted me on the back, and thanked me for getting him a much-needed rest.

I always felt on the outside of any group and never got satisfaction from anything I did. I attended American Legion Boys State in Sacramento but was unsuccessful in being elected governor. I was snide and critical of the boy who was elected, and I was particularly cutting of the members who ran the show.

Church activities came closest to satisfying me. I felt most accepted and appreciated when I was with the MYF crowd. I think the comfort came from being an accepted leader of the group. I never really became an accepted member of any secular high school social groups. Church activities were the only place where I felt that I belonged and could be myself, even though I was very unsure of who that was.

I could "be myself" in these activities since my NPD manifestations appeared to be accepted by my peers, and all that I understood about myself were my NPD manifestations. Specifically, my sense of self-importance was accepted in church activities (NPD #1); my fantasies about success, beauty, love, etc., were acceptable to my friends (NPD #2); my belief that I was "special" was supported (NPD #3); I received the admiration I felt that I required (NPD #4); and my sense of entitlement was reinforced (NPD #5).

In high school, I decided to become a Methodist minister. I went through the necessary steps to preenroll at Boston University School of Theology and attained conscientious objector (CO) draft status by becoming a local preacher in the Methodist Church. At one Methodist retreat on subjects related to faith and belief, a leader confronted me by commenting that I talked a lot about things I didn't understand and hadn't experienced. I was not a reader in those days, and I tried to fake a wisdom I didn't have.

I was never really satisfied with Christianity. I would visit the Vedanta Society's Hollywood Temple and wanted nothing more than to go on a retreat at the Kali Mandir Ashram near Laguna Beach. I was told that I had to read the works of Swami Vivekananda first. Like my Christian critics, the Vedanta crowd also recognized my superficial understanding (NPD #1).

The turbulence and confusion I experienced in high school was apparent to those around me, particularly my teachers. I had an English teacher who was very straightforward with her ideas and feelings.

She put the following comment on one of the papers I handed in: "You seem to be in a continual state of emotional new beginnings."

I remember not reacting to her comment one way or another. The idea was new to me, but it seemed correct.

My NPD was apparent to my family, although they had no name for it in those days. Suzy used to say that I couldn't see beyond my nose. Lack of empathy (NPD #7) was my most conspicuously objectionable NPD characteristic. The father of a neighborhood friend criticized me for not caring about other people. Pop could see the NPD symptoms, and they troubled him. From my early teens, my father would complain that I was "not loving." He was afraid that I would grow up to be a criminal. (When I worked for the Quakers, they too criticized me for not being loving. I could never understand what they were talking about.)

My NPD was the outcome of how I reacted to my home and family environment. My parents did everything they knew to provide a strong and supportive home life. They tried to give me and my siblings every opportunity, though money was often in short supply. They loaned me money, which I never repaid, and they paid my tuition and fees at Pomona College.

It is easy to blame my parents for my NPD. Yes, they created the environment that developed the disorder, but the environmental problems were the result of their disorders and their misunderstanding of reality and not any negative, conscious decisions on their part. In fact, one of the factors that affected the dysfunction was their strong dedication to create the perfect home environment and the perfect parental support to maximize our chances of becoming happy, productive adults. Their hands-on involvement, though, only magnified their own inadequacies and personal dysfunctions. Because of who they were, separately and together, the dysfunctional environment they created was the best they could do.

They were aware that something was wrong before I was. They thought my strange behavior was a medical problem related to the seizures. They may have maintained that opinion forever, but they never discussed it with me. I learned about it from Suzy. When I was undergoing weekly psychotherapy in Washington, DC, I tried to have a face-to-face discussion with my parents about my counseling. In California for a visit, I sat with them in their living room and tried to discuss my concerns about my experiences while growing up. They were defensive and negative about anything psychological and only wanted to talk about how special I was. Pop kept declaring how much he loved me. I believe he did. He glossed over my inability to keep a job and tried to be supportive of the various jobs I'd had. Both parents tried to be there for me, but none of us understood NPD. There was nothing any of us could do to address the problem, much less solve it.

My worldview still told me that I was special and destined to discover a life with no conflict, only happiness and fulfillment. This view did not involve doing anything or achieving anything to warrant this expectation of an ideal existence. Years later, in psychotherapy, I had a persistent illusion that I would eventually walk through an arch and emerge into the ideal world of my imagination. In my later practice of Zen Buddhism, I had the same illusion of some future state of ideal enlightenment. Life was a game in which I was killing time until the great transformation occurred, without any effort on my part. My work, my counseling, my Zen practice, my marriages, and fatherhood—everything in my life—was part of a dream that involved little energy and no emotional feeling or involvement (NPD #1).

It seems clear to me that my NPD, in part at least, was the result of my family experience while I was growing up, prior to leaving home for college in 1953. I was probably more sensitive to positive and negative aspects of my family life than many people would have been, but that was just my genetic makeup. There were clear and present family conflicts that I want to summarize and that I think led to the development of my NPD.

Mother was bright and intellectual but not emotional or truly empathetic. As a teacher, she could be compassionate about her students, and she was compassionate when our dog Judy was hit by a car when I was six. However, she could never understand how people got attached to the movie character ET since he wasn't human. Mother's emotional responses seemed to be preprogrammed, determined or influenced by what people she respected thought or felt.

Mother had strong opinions about everything, and she was deeply critical of Pop. Since he was weak in many ways, she tried to play the supportive role of both mother and father. I have more of my mother's characteristics than my father's. Physically, Mother and I were more alike, and we were more alike in the ways we thought and behaved. I felt closer to Mother than to Pop. When I would come home from college, we would sometimes sit up and talk until after midnight. My father, however, always went to bed at 10 p.m.

Mother, with her strong opinions and expectations, had far more influence on my thinking and behavior than did Pop. She was quite insecure but always wanted to be the "Type A" in any situation without having to admit it. She always wanted people to do what she wanted them to do without having to tell them. She certainly did not want to compete with another woman for my time and affection. She had great difficulty accepting both of my wives; both of them, however, were very insightful about her. Mother probably knew that.

Pop was a different person in every way. Having grown up in a rural, low-income community in upstate New York, he was insecure and, by his own admission, had lots of fears. He was not a strong personality. He was not revered by his parents, unlike his older sister Frances. Pop was not as smart, intellectually or academically, as Mother. He liked to read and became knowledgeable on a number of subjects, but he was not good at studying for exams such as when he tried to become a certified life insurance underwriter. Pop's father had a lot of problems and was not a strong male model. Pop was deeply empathetic and strongly compassionate. He had a profound love for his three children. He was somewhat frightened and put off by my NPD, which he recognized even if he couldn't name it.

When all the facts of my childhood are laid bare, one conclusion stares me in the face: My mother brought me up to be the ideal mate she never had and, as a result, created a person with NPD. She and Pop had little in common, but she and I were similar in many ways. She told me near the end of her life that she was sorry she ever went to that Epworth League meeting in the South Pasadena Methodist Church where she met my father. I think she knew from the start that the relationship wouldn't work, but she had an I-can-fix-anything personality. If he was incapable of being the strong and successful father, she was confident that she could make up for his deficiencies and create the ideal son. Instead of the ideal son, she created a narcissist with a personality disorder.

Both of their lives were sadly pathetic and unsatisfactory, and both were incapable of change. They sought out friends who were wealthy, prominent, or famous, and attempted to achieve through association. Mother outlived all her real friends from high school. Pop did not have any friends; he had acquaintances, some of whom thought highly of him.

Pop wanted to be accepted in the same kind of society that mother came from, but he never got close to being able to play that game. Pop had a good understanding of his dysfunctional family, and he tried to change who he had become as a result of it by moving to California and getting a degree from the University of Southern California. Pop probably realized that Mother regretted marrying him, but there was nothing he could do about it. He said that he married Mother because she had good genes and would bear bright children.

As for being successful, Pop wasn't strong enough to pull it off, and he knew it. Mother came from a dysfunctional family of a different kind, but she could never accept that and always maintained that her childhood was ideal, even though she never spoke of it to us. Pop would always tell Suzy and me stories about his childhood.

I think that Pop wanted to divorce Mother, but he didn't have the courage to consider it seriously. When I was in sixth grade, Pop was very friendly with a woman (Elsie) who worked with the Methodist Church youth program. Because I am virtually certain that he didn't have the guts to proceed, Pop and Elsie never had a sexual relationship as far as I know. I remember feeling at the time that I wished Pop would divorce Mother and marry Elsie.

For as long as he lived, Pop always acted as though he should be awarded a medal for never getting divorced. He could be very embarrassing by commenting at inappropriate times against divorce. He developed a deep attachment against divorce and against people who had gotten divorced, since this is what he wanted to do but never had the strength to even consider it. Had the subject come up, I don't think that Mother would have opposed it. As for myself, I have never been able to emotionally identify with children in novels and movies who were devastated by their parents' divorce or the threat of it. I always openly admitted that I would have welcomed the divorce of Mother and Pop.

It is easy in retrospect to see what a strong influence Mother had on what I thought and on how I behaved in those formative years. I was already manifesting most of the characteristics of NPD, but I was not yet aware of how conflicted and critical I felt about our relationship while I was living at home. When I got to Deep Springs College, I began to examine the conflicts in my mind about who I was and how I got that way.

Deep Springs and Beyond

My Life Changes Dramatically

I was accepted for admission to Whittier College in southern California during my senior year of high school in 1953. I was also selected to have a regional leadership position in the MYF. Then, late in my senior year at Monrovia High School, I was launched into a new chapter that would change my life forever.

A close friend of the family—a professor at the University of California, Los Angeles—was invited to give a lecture at Deep Springs College. While there, he recommended me for admission. I applied and was accepted. That was clearly the most significant occurrence of my life until my second wife Christina successfully confronted me with my NPD 40 years later.

Mother said that she and her father had driven through Deep Springs Valley in 1929 on their way to visit his old hometown in Nevada. When they saw the college, she told my grandfather that she would never let a son of hers go to a school like that. She never changed her mind about the school, but she didn't stop me from going.

Deep Springs College is located in a 43,000-acre, mile-high desert valley in the White Mountains east of Bishop, California. It had a student body of 18 men, who lived and worked at the school; that number has increased to 25 in the last few years. No tuition is charged. The school operates a cattle ranch and farm for the education and experience of the students. Students used to attend for three years, and then transfer to a degree-granting institution as a junior; the stay is now two years. The emphasis was on rigorous academics with a

20-hour work week on the farm and ranch. Founded in 1917, Deep Springs is still vital, well funded, and dynamic. After years of conflict and court action, the board of directors voted to accept women in the student body, and the first ones came in 2018.

In 1953, the Deep Springs administration was at its weakest, but the student body was one of the strongest and most intellectual in its history. Intellectual debate on any subject was a "master or perish" parlor sport. Six faculty members lived on campus with their families, along with the director and his wife. Staff included the mechanic, the ranch manager, the cook, and the cowboy. The student body ran the school and all its operations. The academic program was hands-on and rigorous with frequently only one or two boys in a class.

The school's founder L. L. Nunn said that he created Deep Springs so that a few men could "experience the voice of the desert" and prepare themselves for a life of service to humanity. The school has always been a cloistered experience with restricted contact with the outside world. Students were not allowed to go into town without a student-body leave of absence. In its 100 years of existence, between 1,100 and 1,200 men have attended the college; there are now approximately 700 living alumni.

Most of the Deep Springs students came from prep schools in the East. The SAT average percentile was in the high 90s. Deep Springs graduates could easily transfer to any university of their choice after two or three years; many, if not most, went to the Ivy League. I thrived there and transferred to Pomona College after two and one-half years.

When I entered Deep Springs, I had already investigated several religious traditions. Although I had visited the Vedanta Society in Hollywood on a number of occasions, I was a traditional white, Anglo-Saxon protestant with a Methodist background, a candidate for the ministry, and a CO. After my first year at Deep Springs, I was no longer a believer in God. I was no longer a CO. Instead, I embarked on a lifetime of Zen Buddhist study and practice.

Never before had I felt as comfortable as I did at Deep Springs. I did well academically. I did well on the labor program. I was elected to the highest student body office of labor commissioner. I was also a practical joker. With a couple of friends, I imported some cockroaches from Cuba and put them in the cereal bowls on the dean's table in the dining room. We also put red food dye in the drinking water system, which caused some confusion and much annoyance on the part of faculty and staff. Several friends and I ordered a six-foot iguana from a catalog. We had built a cage in the basement of our main building, and our plan was to ask the director to pick up the package for us at the bus station in Bishop after notification of its arrival. We aborted the plan and cancelled the order when the director nailed me for the cockroaches.

I had a number of significant insights about myself while at Deep Springs. One of the most significant resulted from a conversation with the mechanic Reeve Deason. Reeve and I were out on the desert, repairing a wooden pipe that brought water from a permanent creek in a canyon to the reservoir on campus. I told him I had chosen a pair of cowboy boots that I wanted to buy through a mail-order catalog. I had the money and needed the boots to safely ride the ranch horses, but I couldn't bring myself to write a check and send in the order.

Reeve said, "I'm pretty sure you never made a decision alone before. Am I right?"

He was right. My parents were always there to validate my decision in some way. I had grown up far more sheltered than I realized. Reeve was one of my best teachers at Deep Springs.

Bruce McCully was a Professor Emeritus of English Literature from Pomona College. I took many courses from him at Deep Springs, and he became a major influence on my thinking. He said that students were like pots: Some were clay and broke when you tried to shape them; some were brass that could be pounded into shape.

"You're of the brass variety, Lawrie," he said.

He radically turned my perceptions away from romantic sentimentalism to a more rigorous analytic approach. He taught me how to think. I spent decades thinking about Zen and the teachings of the Buddha before I discovered that the experience of Zen is not accessible through thinking.

My life before Deep Springs was sheltered. My NPD, though it was unknown to me, resulted in much discomfort, but I could not confront my situation. I'll never know how Deep Springs might have affected me had I not been in the throes of NPD. As it was, Deep Springs allowed me to drop all my old values, concepts, and beliefs and begin the long struggle of finding out who I was.

My initial experience with counseling occurred in my first year. I was also introduced to Zen in my first year. I began to discover the deep dysfunction of my family. When I went home for my first visit since entering Deep Springs, I found it very hard to be around my parents, and my best high-school friend and I had nothing to say to each other. Today—66 years after joining the class of '53—the influences, experiences, and permanent changes that Deep Springs represented to me are still present. I had lived with my NPD since early childhood, but it was Deep Springs that opened me to the reality that something was wrong and started me on the long path of finding out what that *something* actually was.

After graduating from Pomona College, I did not maintain contact with Deep Springs. Feeling that my life was unsuccessful, I was embarrassed to remain on the Deep Springs mailing list. It is only in the last 20 years that I have resurfaced as an alumnus.

Two and one-half years at Deep Springs was the only time in my adulthood in which I felt happy and successful and embarked on something meaningful. Deep Springs College affected me deeply because it opened a whole new world for me. I was encouraged by members of the board of directors to leave California and go to Cornell University in Ithaca, New York, where I could live in a fraternity house with other Deep Springs alumni and continue to grow; however, I was frightened by that possibility and opportunity. I stayed stuck and never really emancipated myself from my parents before each had died.

When I was 58 years old, I accepted my NPD, and my life began to change in a positive way. I still feel deeply emotional about Deep Springs and very sad that I was unable to allow Deep Springs to propel me into a life that was not dominated by my attachment to my mother. I was not ready for what might have been, but I was introduced at Deep Springs to Zen, to learning, and to the quest that has brought me to where I am now.

My Introduction to Zen

Alan Watts came to Deep Springs for a weekend of lectures and "hanging out" with the students. Watts was the face of Zen in America in the '50s and '60s. He is still widely read, and his books are still in publication. He introduced me to Zen. We had never heard of him, and we knew nothing about Zen. His very popular book, *The Way of Zen,*[7] was not to be published for three more years. I was instantly enthusiastic about Zen. I think Zen clicked with me because it seemed to provide an immediate window to enlightenment.

Watts was relaxed and friendly, easy to relate to, very human, and charismatic. He was one of those people who appeared to experience the essence of Zen instantaneously, with no process or preparation. He talked about how the world looked from a Zen perspective. He made it seem easy and natural. He was like J. Krishnamurti[8] when he said that there is no way and no path and to just drop the illusions and be enlightened.

I couldn't intellectualize my feelings at the time, of course, since I was not aware of my NPD. However, Zen seemed to be my vehicle to being special. Zen held out the possibility to experience life suddenly, with no conflict, no dread, and no fear. It was the magic archway to the promised land. Alan Watts was there, and I could be there too.

It is now clear to me that Watts was a good spokesperson at that time for a version of Zen that is really not what Zen is understood to be today. It can be tempting to become attached to what Watts is saying in his writing and miss what he is missing. However, Zen goes far more deeply into the reality of emptiness than was portrayed by Watts, and the process of Zen practice is far more difficult and demanding than Watts apparently understood. My understanding of Zen started out and remained for many decades quite superficial. I was not ready for anything deeper because I certainly could have found it if I had been ready.

I now realize that Zen both fueled my NPD and eventually enabled me to drop the illusion that produced it. The person with a Zen practice has the

---

[7] Alan Watts, *The Way of Zen* (New York: Pantheon Books, Inc., 1957).

[8] Jiddu Krishnamurti was an Indian philosopher, speaker, and writer.

possibility of seeing through this illusion ultimately. The person with NPD is stuck with the disorder until they are able to grasp that their life is not working and that they must be open to alternatives. Unfortunately, this almost never happens.

Because of my personal and professional failures, I became open to alternative ways of viewing life and myself. The person with NPD experiences their destructive "self" as the center of the world without realizing that they are doing so. They have created an unconscious distortion of reality, which they are totally incapable of questioning or challenging. The nature and genesis of NPD are such that an openness to alternative understandings of themselves and the world essentially cannot become options.

I previously said that Zen probably fueled my NPD. The person with NPD is going to sit in Zen meditation—zazen[9]—without an intellectual awareness that the concept of a separate and permanent self is an illusion. Unfortunately, many people who are not narcissistic make the same mistake, but there is a greater possibility that they will discover the reality of the "separate self illusion" than does a person with NPD. Also, Zen can provide a person with NPD another opportunity to feel superior and special (NPD #1 and #3). Eventually, however, as I discuss below, Zen was a significant help in my emergence out of NPD.

A Man among Men at Sea

One of the trustees of Deep Springs was a vice president of the Union Oil Company of California. He arranged for Deep Springers to sail on their ships in the summer as extra-Ordinary seamen. We had seaman's papers but were employed in addition to a full union crew, so we were not a threat to the Seaman's Union. I spent the summer of 1954 sailing from Los Angeles and San Francisco to Hawaii.

This was my first experience as a man among men. I got along well with my fellow crewmen and enjoyed getting drunk with them every time we hit port. I will always remember two high points. The first was when I was sitting

---

[9] "Zazen" is formal Zen meditation.

in the mess hall with a cup of coffee and a bad hangover, and I heard a crew-man, who was showing a new seaman around the ship, refer to me as a "regu-lar guy." The other high point was when I was drinking with some shipmates in a bar. Guys from our ship were seated at various tables. I got into an argument with a seaman from another ship. The argument got hot, and we both stood up. Then my shipmates in the bar stood up to defend me, and the other guy left. That was a great feeling.

In the summer of 1956, I went back to sea on a Union Oil tanker. I got tired of going back and forth from California to Hawaii, so I resigned from my job with Union Oil and joined the Military Sea Transportation Service (MSTS) for the 1956 Arctic Expedition to take diesel fuel to the Distant Early Warning (DEW) line radar stations in the Arctic Ocean.

In San Francisco, I went onboard the ship that needed additional crew for the trip to the Arctic and talked to the captain. He told me that he needed expe-rienced seaman and that my experience was not sufficient to fill a slot as an Able-Bodied (AB) seaman. I went directly to the MSTS offices in San Francisco with the papers and qualifications to sign on as an Ordinary seaman. Since they couldn't find any more AB seamen, they gave me a waiver and signed me on as an AB seaman. I went aboard the ship on which I had previously been denied employment and was assigned to the 8-to-12 (morning and nighttime) watch in a stateroom with two roommates—an Ordinary seaman and an AB seaman.

The ship left San Francisco and headed north for Seattle. This stretch of ocean can be some of the roughest in the Pacific. I was seasick from the time we left San Francisco until we entered the Strait of Juan de Fuca, north of Seattle. At 8 a.m., I went to the bridge to take my shift at the helm. The helms-man whom I was relieving asked if I needed any help or advice.

"No," I said, "I can handle it," and took the wheel.

The helmsman gave me the course to steer but did not indicate how strongly the seas were pushing the bow to the right. The waves were terrific, and water flowed all over the foredeck. Not compensating adequately for the pressure of the storm, I was heading too much into the east. Two AB seamen were trying to secure gear on the foredeck when a huge wave washed over them. They stayed onboard, but it was frightening. I was clearly not in control of the ship.

The captain, who had previously turned me down, appeared on the bridge and screamed, "WHAT ARE YOU DOING HERE?"

He threw me off the bridge and promoted the Ordinary seaman on my watch to AB seaman. The next day, I was told that I could take a demotion to Ordinary seaman or be flown back to San Francisco and discharged. I said that I had been looking for a job as an Ordinary seaman in the first place, so I stayed on for the trip north.

We were at sea for six weeks. We sailed north to Point Barrow in Alaska and then east to Cambridge Bay in northern Canada, due north of Kansas City, Missouri. The captain who wouldn't hire me was replaced in Seattle and didn't make the trip. There was no further unpleasantness, but the incident on the bridge was a prime example of my arrogant grandiosity in walking into situations that I couldn't handle while disdaining any help or instruction (NPD #1).

Being an American merchant seaman is very seductive. The food is good, the work is light, you share a stateroom with two other people, and you work only four hours on and eight hours off. If you work during your time off, you get paid overtime. Best of all, the ship is always moving, and you feel as though something is happening and you are going places. Our bosun[10] had shipped out 20 years prior to our trip to supplement his college football scholarship, and he was still sailing.

When we got home, the MSTS asked me to sign on for the Antarctic Expedition.

"No, thanks," I answered. "I'm going back to college."

I didn't want to get seduced into a career at sea like the bosun.

Summer Illusions

During one of the Deep Springs summers, I worked as a program director at country-and-western radio station KXLA in Pasadena when that type of music was gaining popularity in the mainstream.

My job was menial, but I had a press pass and access to tickets. I felt like a big man and met interesting people. Johnny Cash was just emerging from

---

[10] A "bosun" is a boatswain and the senior seaman.

Nashville to Hollywood with his group Luther Perkins and The Tennessee Two and Friend. As a member of the press, I went to his Teenage Queen contests in southern California. I heard Billy Graham at the Rose Bowl and sat close to him in the press section down in front. He was amazing to watch, and his delivery was impressive.

When I went to hear Jerry Lewis at the Hollywood Bowl, a strange thing happened. After the performance, people began to leave before the curtain call. Lewis ran onstage, swinging the microphone over his head and screaming at a woman in the first row who had stood up.

"Hey, lady! What are you doing? Hooking?"

He was clearly angry and not faking it. His negative performance made the papers the next day.

During another summer, I got various jobs in the medical industry. I worked as an ambulance attendant in Pasadena. I had no credentials and no training, but they hired me and wanted me to stay when I quit to return to college. The same summer, I worked as a night attendant at a nursing home with over 100 patients. I spent each night running up and down the corridors with a gurney, changing diapers. When a patient entered into the final minutes or hours before death, they would be wheeled into a room just off the staff coffee lounge. Staff could then hear when they had stopped groaning and gasping. I told myself that if anyone started to die on my watch, I would call an ambulance. I don't know who would have paid or what they would have done with a dying patient when they got to the hospital, but no one died on my watch.

The other job I had that summer was a private attendant to a wealthy, middle-aged quadriplegic. He was cynical and snide to others but pleasant enough to me. He had an attractive wife who, in Lady Chatterley fashion, seemed to have a secret arrangement with a man who could meet her needs. It amazes me now how conventional and moralistic I was in those days.

Pomona College

I finished up at Deep Springs in spite of the director—a pathetic character who was not respected by anyone, including the board of directors. He tried to get rid of me and one of my friends after our second year. The board disagreed, not willing to throw up their hands and abandon a couple of young men even if their creativity included troublemaking. The board intervened to allow us to come back for our final year, with my friend as president of the student body and me as labor commissioner. We both left after the first semester of our third year. I don't remember where he went; I went to Pomona College.

Pomona College was a strange experience. I had no reason to be there except to graduate, and I had no idea what I was going to do after that. Those were the days when many people felt that four years of college were necessary just to live life, not to get a meal ticket. I had friends at Deep Springs; however, as I said previously, I didn't keep in touch with anyone after I left. The same was true for Pomona except that, after I graduated, I contacted my best friend once. No one contacted me from either Deep Springs or Pomona. I just didn't bond well with other people.

I majored in English and creative writing, and then switched to philosophy and finally back to English literature. I changed my major several times and had to stay an extra semester to earn enough units in my major to graduate. I was constantly searching for some meaning to hang on to. When I took courses in religion or philosophy, I always looked for possible significance for my life rather than a pure intellectual analysis. Everything felt temporary and in flux.

I would walk across the quad, kicking the leaves and saying to myself, "This isn't going to last long, so I had better enjoy it."

I took all the creative writing classes at Pomona College. Kris Kristofferson, who was in one of my classes, was an outstanding writer even then. I remember one of his stories about a natural rock formation that looked like a bare-chested woman. The community went through a big hassle to get the rock breasts covered with a shroud. Kris was a big man on campus, but my friends and I thought he was kind of stiff and strait-laced; we identified as a bunch of drunken intellectuals who didn't like each other very much.

I had a girlfriend with whom I had my first sexual experience. After a semester in France, she came home a lesbian. I was never a good lover. My mother was the sex education teacher in the family; I never got any instruction from Pop. She overdid her enthusiasm for enjoyable sex—no doubt this was

38

because she never had any. Nevertheless, she had strong ideas about how sexuality should be expressed. To her, foreplay and intercourse were irrelevant. All that mattered was that sex should be with a permanent mate with whom you were deeply in love.

Mother's strong ideas and my lack of empathy were clearly the causes of my inability to be a good lover. I was told that I didn't make love; I just ignored my partner for my own pleasure. However, I was never interested in "sex for sex." I was looking for something more, a "mountaintop experience," which I never found.

My crass selfishness as a lover and pursuer of women is daunting to remember. I totally objectified the women with whom I had intercourse. I never had an ongoing extramarital relationship after I married; however, I was a one-event fornicator from time to time but never had an overnight experience with any of my conquests. I was neither a sensitive lover of my wives nor a caring lover in my infidelities. I was not violent or physically exploitative; I was just never "there," never concerned about the woman's experience. My sexual experience was a clear expression of my NPD. (It might be interesting to note that my brother Don's wife commented to me once that he was a lousy lover because of Mother's influence on him.)

While at Pomona, I had some therapy sessions with a psychologist and thought that I wanted to discuss my girlfriend. It quickly became obvious that I was there to talk about myself. After a few sessions, the psychologist told me that I would never be hospitalized for my problems, but I would probably have a history of feeling dissatisfied with what I was doing and leave job after job for something I might like better.

It was clear in my mind that I didn't want an ordinary job and "a house in the suburbs with a dog and a white picket fence." I didn't know what I wanted. My psychologist didn't know how to name or define my problem, but he was right in his diagnosis. NPD was not included in the first DSM published in 1952. This was only the beginning of my long trek through the world of mental health, seeking some answer to the unrest and discontent I felt and the key to emerging into a world of peace.

Into the World of Men and Women

I finished my studies at Pomona in early 1959. I didn't know what I wanted to do next, but I thought I ought to go to graduate school to avoid the draft. I took the Graduate Record Exam and didn't do well. I was angry at the dean of students at Pomona for telling me that there was no point in taking the exam over, that I would just have to live with the score I had, and that it wouldn't change if I took it again. I didn't believe him, but I was afraid to set myself up for another failure.

I had no goals or expectations about graduate school or a profession. My parents always encouraged me to get a PhD degree. This was possibly good advice, but I always thought it was because they wanted a PhD in the family and not because they thought it would be good for me. Both were probably true.

I applied for Officer Candidate School and was accepted. Prior to reporting for duty in the navy, I looked up a professor who taught Zen at Claremont Graduate University. Although I considered myself a Zen Buddhist and had read a lot of books on the subject, I had not yet been taught how to do Zen meditation. That was not part of Alan Watts's introduction.

After talking to me for a while, the Claremont professor said, "Stop studying Zen! You're too glib," and suggested that I go into the navy and just vegetate. "Zen is like a blind rat in a dark corner. Zen takes the gun from the soldier and food from a starving man."

His advice was to just go and hang out. I went into the navy but ignored everything he told me.

The navy inadvertently showcased my disorder. I made it through Officer Candidate School without distinction and got commissioned. Within the first hour of my commissioning, I was harassing senior noncommissioned officers for failing to salute. I went home on leave, impressed with my new status as an ensign, and wore my uniform home, although that was not required.

I requested a noncombatant ship and was assigned to the refrigerator supply ship USS *Rigel*. We carried supplies from various ports in the United States and Europe to ships in the Mediterranean Sea. It was good duty—easy and fun. I could have had a great time for three years if I had been able to relax, carry out my duties, and play tourist in Europe.

However, I was not good at leisure. I brought a lot of books on board, none of them novels or travel books. Against the professor's advice, I continued to devour Zen and philosophy. I went to the First Zen Institute of America in New York in 1960 and learned to do Zen meditation. I have done zazen daily ever since, with long and short breaks, but consistently since the 1980s. I read and meditated while I was a naval officer. I socialized little and developed no close friendships.

At ports of call in Europe and the Caribbean, I did some obligatory sightseeing, but mostly I drank and scouted out women and usually paid for sex with them. I got my first and only case of gonorrhea from a woman in Palma de Mallorca, who introduced me to paella. I paid for the paella but not for the sex.[11]

I was sent to Newport, Rhode Island, to attend Law Officer School and Cryptanalysis School. Still insecure and unfulfilled, I was seeking something, and Zen was not giving me answers. The Newport facility housed a number of schools, and Naval Chaplaincy School and Center was one. I befriended a young priest at the school and told him about my psychological discomforts and Zen studies. He thought I was disturbed and suggested that I see the base psychiatrist. Oddly enough, I did.

---

[11] The memory of gonorrhea has thankfully not spoiled my continuing taste for paella: a Spanish dish of rice, saffron, chicken, and seafood, stewed and served in a large shallow pan.

The navy pulled me out of school and put me in Sick Officers Quarters. I saw a psychiatrist every day and told him about my seizure history. The navy tested me, and then took me off the medication I had been taking sporadically. I no longer had a brain abnormality, and I hadn't had a seizure for nearly 10 years. I thought I might get a medical discharge and liked the idea the more I thought about it. Finally, the doctor pronounced that I was in good shape and was sending me back to duty.

The doctor wrote in my medical file, "Although Ensign White has a profound dislike for the military and a history of pacifism, he is an above average Naval Officer and is returned to full active duty."

I finished classes and was certified as a law officer and a crypto officer. Back onboard ship, no sooner had I moved into an empty, single-bed stateroom than I was ordered out by the executive officer and put in a double with another ensign. The exec didn't seem to understand that I was entitled (NPD #5).

My ship was anchored in the Bay of Naples, Italy. The liberty boat was full of enlisted personnel, waiting at the bottom of the loading ladder for a duty officer to come aboard so that they could go ashore on leave. I was the duty officer. In winter blue uniform, including great coat, I came down the ladder. At the bottom was a float to which the liberty boat was tied and against which it was bobbing up and down in moderately rough seas.

I descended the ladder onto the float, stepped across the float, and attempted to step into the boat. Instead, I stepped into the water between the boat and the float. Someone grabbed my hair and pulled me aside as the boat banged violently into the float. Pulled from the water, unhurt but drenched, I faced the boat full of somber men who had almost witnessed a death by crushing.

I turned to the senior petty officer and said, "That must have looked ridiculous. You may give these men permission to laugh."

I slopped up the ladder and entered the ship. The sailors were deadly silent until I closed the hatch, and then they broke into gales of laughter. I changed out of my dress blues and returned to my duties. You can be sure I watched my step the second time down.

On another occasion, we were steaming in the Mediterranean when we were suddenly being harassed by Russian ships crossing our bow. I was standing watch on the bridge as officer of the deck. My orders were to maintain course and speed, even if that meant plowing into one of the Russian vessels. I decided that the order was stupid and could get someone killed, so I determined to alter course and avoid a collision if the situation arose; fortunately, it never did.

My arrogance in being willing to disobey direct orders was based on the idea that I knew better than my seasoned superiors (NPD #9). I was serious about how important my position was, but I didn't really take my job seriously. I also didn't take relationships seriously. I never felt that I belonged. It was as though I was acting in a play or having a dream. Everything seemed temporary and on the brink of disaster. My naval career came to an end, but these feelings did not.

Restless and uncomfortable, I wanted something to make everything right. It wasn't going to happen onboard ship. I had been looking forward to a medical discharge; since that possibility was over, I decided to look into resigning as a CO. I contacted the office of the American Friends Service Committee (AFSC), which had a full-time person helping people attain CO status. I submitted the papers and was given an interview with the captain who headed the chaplain service on the East Coast.

The captain and I met in his office in Norfolk, Virginia, and had an interesting debate. He maintained that I had a contract to fulfill. I countered that the contract was immoral and therefore invalid. I won the debate and took home the prize of an honorable discharge. I suspect that no one regretted my leaving. The navy handled this incident professionally and without apparent prejudice or emotion. I, on the other hand, was willing to use any Jesuitical ruse to win my appeal, including Christian arguments and biblical references in which I did not believe, even as I professed to be a Zen Buddhist as my dog tags claimed.

When I got out in 1960, the Friends Committee on National Legislation (FCNL)—the Quaker political lobby that supported my departure from the navy—offered me a job as their fundraiser. I rented an apartment (in a building where John Philip Sousa had lived) near the FCNL offices on Capitol Hill in Washington, DC. I traveled the country in a new car, visiting Quaker meetings and individual Quakers from Massachusetts to North Carolina to Ohio.

The FCNL was my first real civilian job. It could have been easy and fulfilling, but it wasn't long before people began to question why I wasn't more loving, echoing my father's criticism. Compassion and concern for justice and civil rights are the heart and marrow of the FCNL, but I couldn't see devoting my career to it. I may have been out of sync with their mission, but they appreciated my work.

I went to John F. Kennedy's inauguration and nearly froze to death, standing on the grass very close to the podium. When I could no longer stand the cold, I went home to watch the rest of the ceremonies on television. After Kennedy took up residence in the White House, I frequently picketed the place during my lunch hour. We in the Peace Movement were working to ban atmospheric atomic testing. The camaraderie of this protest movement was a good vehicle for an NPD sufferer to attain some recognition and attention.

I met my future wife Willo while she was working at the Washington International Student Center. She arranged for several of the students and me to meet Bobby Kennedy in his office. Byron White, who later became a Supreme Court justice, was in the office at the time. We talked briefly, concluding that we were probably not related. Bobby was a slight, slender man with a big smile and a lock of hair falling across his forehead. Both men were cordial, and the conversations were brief.

Willo and I received frequent invitations to embassy parties in Washington because of our jobs. One of the parties at the Soviet Embassy was expertly hosted by Soviet Ambassador Anatoly Dobrynin, who was charming as he circulated to speak with everyone, including us. At the same party, Adlai Stevenson II, Ambassador to the United Nations, was pleasant and approachable, but I was shocked at how fat he had become. I didn't see him once without a plate of food in his hands.

After most of the guests had left, Willo and I got into a conversation with a young Russian couple—a second secretary or something. I had been drinking Russian vodka for the first time and was getting drunker and drunker. I had only ever drunk the medicinal American version, but this stuff went down like water. We were also diving into the smoked salmon and Beluga caviar. We were all laughing and having a lot of fun. Both women remained reasonably sober, so they could drive us home. I got drunk enough to make the grand announcement that if the communists would assure the rights of the individual, I would join the Communist Party. We made it home all right, and we never saw the couple again.

I had lunch with senior officers from the Soviet Embassy from time to time.

One day at lunch with several Soviets, the first secretary turned to me and asked, "What is the John Birch Society?"

I told him that it was the most conservative of the American far-right organizations.

On another occasion, several New York Quakers, who were Wall Street brokers, wanted me to put together a lunch in Washington with some genuine Soviet communists. The guests were several Soviets, including the first secretary of the embassy, and three Quaker stockbrokers. They got along famously and discovered that they were all playing the same game: power and control. I was the odd man out: a far-left intellectual liberal, a mere idealist. The Soviets and the Wall Street Quakers agreed that what I was preaching was too radical and I should be put in prison if I voiced my opinions in public. I think their reaction was because I sounded like a communist or a revolutionary at a time when the country was very sensitive about far-left speech.

I enjoyed making people uncomfortable, which was clearly a result of my feelings of inadequacy. I enjoyed the thought that I probably had a negative file at the FBI because I was one of the people who picketed the CIA after the Bay of Pigs fiasco. The CIA was still in Washington, DC, in those days, and Allen Dulles was the director.

Willo and I became engaged in 1961. Attractive and fun, she had grown up in California and had also gone to Pomona College where her father was a famous professor. I had not known her there, but we seemed to have a lot in common. I was an example of the comment attributed to Pearl Buck: "When it's time to get married, you find the best available partner and do so." We enjoyed each other, and it was a good match. I wasn't capable of truly falling in love, but I asked her to marry me and she accepted.

After our engagement, I was asked to join the crew of the sailboat that had cruised and would again cruise into the Bikini Atoll hydrogen bomb test range to stop the testing. This was a difficult period for us because Willo and I felt that, if I went to the South Pacific, I would not return and marry her. However, this was not because I would be injured but because it would be a life-changing and course-altering experience from which there would be no way back.

I was asked to be navigator on the voyage. I knew I wasn't competent to do it (not that incompetence had ever stopped me before), but I was also hesitant about taking on new experiences away from home. While at the FCNL, I had been asked to consider going to Addis Ababa, Ethiopia, to manage the office of the organization fighting apartheid in South Africa. That was too extreme for me, and I declined. I was timid about new, strange, unknown, and faraway things and places, so I stayed home and we got married in 1962.

Willo and I found a picturesque church outside of Washington for the wedding and had the reception at the home of Willo's father and stepmother in Bethesda, Maryland. We didn't invite anyone who lived outside of the Washington area. Willo went along with this plan, but the idea was mine and I felt strongly about it. It was clearly one of my NPD manifestations, lacking empathy for the feelings of friends and family who would have liked to attend and who were hurt and offended that they were not invited.

My parents would have loved to be included; my plan was in large part to exclude them. I was again overcome by the feeling that what I was doing was not real, permanent, or okay. It felt like a weekend experience that I didn't want to take seriously. A photograph of Willo and me coming down the aisle after the exchange of vows shows me with a distinct "Oh, shit!" expression on my face. I was not capable of making a loving marriage commitment. NPD is like a metastasizing cancer that quietly affects everything you think or do. "Me" becomes a filter through which everything is viewed (NPD #7 and #9).

Willo and I decided to quit our jobs after the wedding and move to Boston, so that I could get a PhD degree. I thought that, with a doctorate, I could become an important leader in the Peace Movement, which seemed always to be growing. I was accepted with a full scholarship at Boston University School of Theology as a PhD candidate in social ethics.

My parents frequently suggested that I get a PhD degree in something, and now I was going to do so. As I said before, my parents attempted to achieve through affiliation, and I think they wanted to be the parents of a doctor because it would make them look good as parents. In spite of it all,

I do think that my parents were concerned about me and knew that I was troubled. I think it was their opinion that I could navigate my way through life with greater satisfaction if I had a graduate degree.

On Labor Day in 1962, we left my parents' house in California and drove to Boston to begin my graduate studies. No sooner had I arrived than I was dissatisfied with graduate school. Did I only want a PhD degree to become a big shot in the Peace Movement? Was it to impress my parents? What was I doing at Boston University when I should be across the river at Harvard?

Willo's friend and coworker in the Admissions Office of the School of Theology invited us that winter to spend a weekend with her and her husband in their traditional stone house in the country. He was an intellectual conversant in all kinds of offbeat subjects. They had a big fireplace with a roaring fire, and the walls were solid bookshelves full of books. We were supposed to come out on Friday and leave on Sunday afternoon. I was so threatened by the ambiance of this home and the subjects discussed that I insisted we leave on Saturday morning. We never saw them again. I don't recall what I found so threatening, but I was naïve and more conventional than I would admit. It was as though new ideas threatened my entire worldview and perhaps the fortress of my disorder.

For people as frightened, confused, and insecure as I was, ideas can be more threatening than physical violence. For those who are truly aware, however, there is a simplicity and beauty about everything, and nothing is threatening. The very presence of people who are truly aware can be a threat to those who are confused and insecure. I found our host and hostess for that weekend terrifying. As I think back on this experience, there was no one thing that triggered my response. I think my fear was that my host was likely to introduce me to ideas and concepts that were threatening to my understanding of who I was and what I believed.

In October 1962, during the Cuban Missile Crisis, we didn't have television, so we were glued to the radio. We were close enough to Logan Airport to hear the military planes taking off. I was concerned about the threat of nuclear war. Although I had voted for Kennedy and considered myself a liberal, the bloom was off the rose, and I was disillusioned with his presidency. I was not in any way a communist or a supporter of Russia, but I had more faith in

Khrushchev avoiding war than in Kennedy doing so. I got so far behind in my Greek language class that I dropped it.

During a conference with my Old Testament professor, a close friend stuck his head in the door and exclaimed, "They murdered Kennedy! Those goddamned John Birchers!"

A number of us sat shiva[12] that night at the home of a Jewish friend. We were all convinced that the John Birch Society was behind the assassination. It was amazing to be in Boston when this happened. Stores closed and people on the street were weeping openly. I was fascinated by the drama but not devastated by the loss.

I was temperamentally conservative and frightened about ideas or concepts that challenged my worldview. For example, when Richard Nixon was pardoned by Gerald Ford, I was mind-blown. I was under the illusion that there was something absolute about the law. I thought it applied to everyone.

When Nixon was pardoned, I thought, "The law is just a game. It depends on all kinds of subjective circumstances."

It was one of my first insights into the reality that nothing is absolute except change, the speed of light, and some physics and mathematical concepts. My parents had tried to shield me from anything unpleasant or controversial. Movies were screened as I was growing up. That's why, at an early age, I used to rebel by saying things I knew would make people uncomfortable, like the elementary schoolteacher in San Gabriel whom I made cry by commenting about her husband in the war. I think that my motivation was not to hurt the teacher per se but to say something outrageous. I would make inappropriate comments at family dinners and similar occasions just to shatter the status quo. I think this was a manifestation of my deep-seated anger. I didn't feel that I could rebel openly.

I was frequently overwhelmed with anxiety attacks regarding death. It wasn't death itself that terrified me. It was the fear of "not being." It was too horrible to contemplate the idea that I, myself, me, would cease to exist. This was of course directly related to my disorder. Although it was certainly not yet clear to me, I was struggling with the illusion of a separate self.

---

[12] "Sitting shiva" is one of the five stages of mourning in Judaism.

I was deeply troubled because I was existentially attached to the "self" that I thought was me and was special. This deep attachment to the idea of a permanent and "special" self is at the heart of NPD. It is also the motivating energy for religion. Religions, however, have come up with answers, "paths," and processes to answer the questions regarding human mortality and purpose. Some of these "answers" are more popular than others. For the person with NPD, the "self" is absolute, permanent, and the only reality, and to question this is deeply disturbing.

The bursar at the School of Theology—a Quaker—conscripted some of the students to preach at Quaker churches on Sundays. These were Protestant Quakers, not the silent-meeting type. In my sermons, I always emphasized the need for an epiphany, which manifested my continuing struggle to find "the answer." This theological approach got me into trouble because these Quakers were used to a less confrontational worldview.

Over the years, I had several involvements with the Religious Society of Friends, always with the silent-meeting or Philadelphia persuasion. The silent-meeting Friends are not necessarily Christian; many members identify theologically with Hinduism or Buddhism. I maintained a Buddhist orientation while associated with the Friends. I have always felt that spiritual practice needed to involve a transformation of awareness or epiphany if one were to develop spiritually.

My problem with the Friends was that their community service and political activity always seemed to take precedence over silence and spirituality. Zen, on the other hand, was direct, with no distractions. For the same reason, I was never attracted to the emphasis of some Zen groups on community service and social engagement. I realize that, for many people, community engagement is at the heart of spiritual practice. It was probably an indication of my NPD that I found personal transformation more compelling than community empathy.

In the summer of 1963, Willo and I volunteered to work for the AFSC in Guatemala. We drove to the regional office of the AFSC in Mexico City. A couple in Boston asked us to drive their car to Mexico City so they could use it while attending a conference. When my parents heard what we were doing for the summer, they volunteered to work in the Mexico City office of the AFSC.

I found this decision annoying, but there was nothing that I could do about it. From Mexico City, we flew to Guatemala.

The Guatemala experience was fun. I enjoyed being called "Don Lorenzo." We broke the AFSC rules by buying a baby goat for a pet. It was undoubtedly stolen by the man who sold it to us and barbequed shortly after we left. We supervised a group of volunteers who were digging latrines for the local community. All of our volunteers had a good time. At the end of the summer, we flew back to Mexico City and drove our friend's car north. We knew about the upcoming Martin Luther King, Jr. gathering in Washington and drove hard to hear him deliver what turned out to be the "I Have a Dream" speech, but we didn't make it in time.

In my second year of graduate school, Willo became pregnant, so I dropped out of school and found a job. The Commonwealth of Massachusetts started a war-on-poverty program before the federal program was initiated, and I was one of the first employees. All kinds of strange jobs were opening up with the new funds available. (I turned down one unbelievable job because it was too unstructured. The Massachusetts government wanted to pay me to drink in the working-class bars around Boston and learn what was bothering people and what needed to be improved to make them happy and productive!) As for my job, I can't remember what I was supposed to be doing. I met with people out of the office a lot.

Alexandra was born in Boston on January 7, 1965. Willo felt strongly about having the delivery with no anesthesia and wanting me in the delivery room, so we launched a search for an obstetrician who would accommodate our requirements. This task demanded face-to-face interviews with a number of doctors before we found one who was happy to comply with our desires. All went well, and we began our family with a beautiful, healthy girl. Looking back on the experience, the difficulty of finding a doctor who was open to what is now standard procedure seems strange.

One of the doctors we interviewed said, "If you want pain, I can give you lots of that."

We passed on him.

My Anger and Rage

The movie *Bonnie and Clyde* had just been released, and people were discussing its overt violence. My boss thought that I was the most violent person he had ever met. This was a shock to me, but it wouldn't have been a surprise to my family. I was deeply angry and raging, but I was not aware of it. I later had several public rage attacks.

One incident was at an airport ticket counter when I couldn't upgrade my ticket to first class because there were no seats available. I made such a scene that another passenger in line offered me his first-class seat and I accepted. The ticket agent seemed relieved to resolve the issue and get rid of me.

The other incident took place at the T-Group (Therapy Group) summer event at the university in Bethel, Maine. This weeklong event was the thing to attend if you were involved in therapy or counseling. Everyone was assigned to a primary group and to breakout groups, and a PhD psychologist was leading the breakout group I attended. Something triggered me, and I went into a blue rage. I don't remember what the trigger was. My anger was so violent that the therapist said he couldn't handle me and left the group. I was devastated to be so successfully powerful. Fortunately, my main group was led by a competent psychologist from the Tavistock Institute in London. He and my main group got me back on an even keel. Until then, I had not been fully aware of my anger. I have never been aware of the core of my anger or what triggered it. I was always somewhat aware of a free-floating anger in the background of my consciousness, but the triggers of specific outbursts were never clear to me.

My family, however, knew my anger and the power of my nonempathetic personality. My father had been inactive with chronic obstructive pulmonary disease for some time, spending his days in a chair in the living room. Mother didn't think he was doing all he should to get better. He had a hard time breathing. She took him to the hospital where they put him on oxygen. He was happy and comfortable the first night, but by morning he had stopped breathing and they had to intubate him.

My sister called and told me that they could not remove the respirator because his heart stopped when they tried to do so. I called the hospital and talked to the attending physician. He told me that they had asked my father if they could remove the tube and he had said no, he didn't want it removed. I said I was coming right out to see him, and the doctor said they could keep him alive until I got there. I drove from Albuquerque to my parent's home in Seal Beach, California. When I arrived, I was told that they had removed the respirator and my father was dead. I erupted in a tantrum and got in the car to drive back to Albuquerque. I screamed all the way to Barstow. I was angry at them for killing my father, and I was angry at Pop for being a loser.

I learned the whole story sometime later, and it was a significant indicator of my disorder. My mother, Suzy, and my son Geoff were in the hospital waiting room when they decided that, if I was coming, they'd better get on with removing the respirator. My mother knew that there was a signed health directive at home that specified nonresuscitation, so they pulled the tube before I got there.

Here is the important point: They were afraid that I would arrive and convince the doctor not to remove the respirator, and then go home and leave my mother and sister to deal with an intubated patient. They did not feel that they could reason with me or that I would be understanding or helpful, regardless of my mother's wishes and the signed document that made the removal appropriate and legal.

In hindsight, I think that I would have agreed to "pull the plug." There was really no alternative, but I can understand my family's unwillingness to trust that I would agree with their decision. Had I been there when he died, I'm sure that I would have felt terrible. Pop was a loving guy and I loved him. I also hated him for being so professionally unsuccessful and for not being there for me all my life. I really think that he tried to be a good father. It would have been very hard to watch him die, particularly after he had asked the doctors not to have the tube removed. The attending doctor told me this information on the phone before I left New Mexico.

The Adult Manifestation

The Dance Goes On

I manifested "a grandiose sense of self-importance" my whole life (NPD #1). I took temporary and permanent jobs for which I wasn't qualified—from a commercial moving van driver to the chief executive officer (CEO) of a behavioral health hospital. I was always much better in the interview than I was in executing the job once I got it. I never prepared for any job I ever held. I always stepped into positions that were new to me and learned on the job. Beneath the grandiosity and self-importance, feelings of insecurity and "not belonging" always existed.

When the War on Poverty got underway nationally in the early '60s, a friend from Boston University put me in touch with a new company that was contracted by the Office of Economic Opportunity (OEO). The University Research Corporation (URC) in Washington, DC, had a contract in Roanoke, Virginia, and I went to work for them to supervise a Community Action Program (CAP). It was a strange job. I didn't really have anything to do.

Willo stayed in Boston, and I moved in with Bristow, the director of the program, and his wife and daughters. I felt right at home and acted like a member of the family, much to the annoyance of Bristow's family (NPD #1 and #7). Soon Willo and Alex joined me, and we rented a house in a neighborhood dominated by white railroad retirees.

After we had been there a few months, we threw a party for the staff of the CAP, which was mostly black. Racial tensions were running high in mid-'60s rural Virginia. Guests parked on the street and walked up the long flight of stairs to the front porch. With a tub of iced drinks and a table of food on the porch, the party got underway with about 20 people. Integrated parties were uncommon, so it was fairly stiff and low key.

Suddenly, the cops mounted the front steps. The police were very professional, polite, and apologetic. The neighbors had seen a caravan of black people on their street descending on our house. We were not doing anything illegal, but the police wanted to keep the neighborhood peace, so they suggested that we move the party to the backyard and keep our front door closed. They helped us move the tub of ice and the table of food around back. This episode brought a dull party to life, and we all proceeded to have a great time.

Geoffrey was born in Roanoke on December 2, 1966. His delivery was without problems, and I was present in the delivery room. When Willo got back to her room in the hospital, I smuggled up some beers so we could celebrate.

Our tenure in Roanoke was coming to an end. The staff of the CAP became concerned that they were not being paid enough and objected to some of Bristow's policies and procedures. I sided with the staff and encouraged the revolt. When Bristow realized that I was involved, he demanded that I leave. We returned to DC, but the URC kept me on their payroll. They basically agreed with my criticism of the Roanoke CAP leadership, even though they felt I had overstepped my role.

Another company offered to pay me more money for doing the same thing—getting and running contracts for the War on Poverty—and thus becoming the URC's competition. I left the URC because I felt that I was more valued and appreciated by the other company and not for the money.

The owners of the URC—a psychiatrist and a PhD sociology professor— saw me as a fellow professional whom they trusted to function independently to bring in governmental contracts. I was well known and respected at the OEO and could have been successful. However, my insecurity made me afraid to function on my own. I was afraid of my own success. The rival company saw my strength and my weakness, providing not only more money but more emotional support. The URC didn't realize how needy and insecure I really was, so I had to leave before they found out. My fear of failure and need for support were always just below the surface, and I always gravitated toward the "safe" rather than the "adventurous" or "independent" alternatives.

The new company set up shop. The president ran the finances, and I got the contracts, hired the staff, and supervised the operations. We were very successful. I was well liked in the OEO, and they offered us money without dictating where we would spend it. We did work for various CAPs around the country during our initial year, and there were two serious problems, both NPD related.

The first problem was that I was good at writing contracts, but I was a terrible administrator, unable to relate to the professional staff I had hired. When we weren't in the field, I hid in my office and wrote proposals.

The other problem was that the president and I were not flexible with our clients. The president had been in the defense contracting business, and his attitude was "no prisoners." Between the two of us, clients' requests for contract changes and operational flexibility didn't have a chance. He and I were deaf to the human and company needs of the people who got the money from the War on Poverty to pay us.

We had a financially successful first year, so we applied to the War on Poverty for a whole range of second-year projects. When project recipients were announced, we were not among them. We fired everyone and went out of business; however, the URC is still in business, and I could have stayed with them indefinitely if not for my disorder (NPD #1, #5, #6, and #7).

I did independent contracting for a few months until a new position fell in my lap. The National Institute of Mental Health (NIMH) had an opportunity to get some War on Poverty money from the Department of Labor if they could commit it by the end of the fiscal year, which was in three months. I was hired by the NIMH as a temporary GS-15[13] to put together a staff and commit $3 million in three months to various CAPs. I supervised the spending of that money over the next two years. Our task was to give each of the CAPs that we had selected as much money as they could spend in a year to increase low-income citizen participation in their programs.

---

[13] "GS-15" is a General Schedule employee at the highest civil-service level and paygrade.

After we had given the CAPs the money, we came back to check on them from time to time and conducted weekend training workshops. The workshops usually concluded with a party and heavy drinking. Some of the training sessions were unbelievably presumptuous. During one weekend, we held a meeting in a conference hotel in Harpers Ferry, West Virginia. I told about 25 trainees—black and white—that a training exercise would happen. I did not tell them that the room we were using was wired, so that we could record their reactions.

While I was talking, by prearrangement, one of my staff came in and whispered something in my ear. He left, and I explained to the group that the hotel administration asked that all the black trainees move out of the main building and into the cabins around the campus. I left the room, and we taped the responses for about 30 minutes. Even though I had told the group that this was a training exercise, most of them didn't interpret the situation that way.

Their reactions were predictably strong. Several black trainees, deeply scandalized, said that they quit the job for which they were supposedly being trained. I came back after 30 minutes and explained that it had been part of the training. We discussed the experience, and some insights even emerged. Some welcomed the opportunity to get in touch with their feelings.

This thoughtless and inconsiderate stunt was my idea, a grandiose indulgence. We were lucky that everyone took it well and no one assaulted us (NPD #1, #5, #6, #7, and #9—a royal flush of disorder).

My two-year adventure with the War on Poverty was a case study in both NPD and government waste. I hired several staff members who were temporary GS-12s. One female staff member lived and worked in San Francisco, so we got together at least once a month on one coast or the other. We used to carry pot in our briefcases on the plane. Once, when she was rushing to catch a flight in Dulles International Airport, her briefcase flew open and baggies of pot littered the terminal floor. She blithely scooped them up and continued on her way, unmolested.

When the program began, I had put together an administrative budget that I assumed would be evaluated and reduced. It wasn't, so I had all the excess I'd asked for. From time to time, I shared my expense-account money with my supervisor, who had a mistress in his division, by allowing him to use some of my travel money for his staff. At a conference in South Carolina, the mistress was there, but our boss was not. I stupidly came on to her, and she responded in a passive and provocative way. Nothing else happened, but I assumed that she told my boss about my inept pass and eliminated my chances of staying on with the NIMH (NPD #5 and #2).

Arthur Janov lived in Beverly Hills and had recently published his book, *The Primal Scream*.[14] His method of therapy was supposed to cure all of one's neuroses instantly. He had sold a million copies, and The Beatles had gone through his therapy program. This was my kind of program for instant enlightenment!

I got in touch with Janov, and we met at his office in Beverly Hills. He wanted me to get him an NIMH grant to legitimize his primal-scream therapy. I wanted him to put me through his $20,000+ program for free. He was open to the proposition if I could produce from the NIMH side, which of course I couldn't do. We hung out for a full day, trying to con each other. He won. I agreed to set up a presentation for him at the NIMH and fly him and his wife to Washington first class. He did not agree to put me through his program. I scheduled a large auditorium at the NIMH with a full house to be followed by a smaller, more intimate meeting that would be by invitation only. I invited my current therapist Shelly Kopp, who was annoyed because he thought the "intimate" gathering was too large.

While I was in California meeting with Janov, I ran across the dean of a school of professional psychology that offered a PsyD degree. This dean wanted me to set up a program in Washington, DC, where I and several other people could obtain PsyD degrees. I found an attractive woman who wanted to be part of the program and was qualified. All was going well except that, in the final interviews in California, I kept raving about Janov and *The Primal Scream* being the last words in clinical psychology. These administrators decided that I wasn't the person they were looking for and terminated plans for a Washington program (NPD #1, #2, #4, and #5).

Ever-present fantasies of success always dominated the ever-present fear of failure. This was true in the bedroom as well as in the boardroom. Fantasies

---

[14] Arthur Janov, *The Primal Scream* (New York: Dell Publishing, 1970).

of ideal love destroyed my enjoyment of sex. Fantasies of success in the corporate or nonprofit worlds destroyed my ability to do the work in front of me or to make the social sacrifices that lead to true success. My fantastic belief in being "special," developed by my mother, was not so much a conscious idea as it was the permanent background noise accompanied by a basic feeling of inadequacy.

Fantasies of universal admiration were actually a cowering need for approval.

Performing the duties of a caring father in a well-functioning family was not something that I did well nor is it really possible for a person with NPD. In the late '60s, when Willo, Alex, Geoffrey, and I were living in Washington, DC, we took a vacation to Virginia Beach just after Labor Day when it was still warm and enjoyable but the crowds were gone.

I remember lying on the beach with Willo and our two kids. The temperature was perfect, and the beach was deserted. There were so many things we could have done together. Everyone was soaking up the sun and enjoying being together as a family—everyone except me. Everything I did with my time and life was related to me and my drives, desires, and fantasies. I was incapable of thinking of what was good, fun, or right for the family. In fact, I was no good at having fun by myself, much less with other people.

Restless and uncomfortable, I didn't know how to just hang out and enjoy my wife and kids. The discomfort got so strong that I left everyone at the beach, flew home to DC, and searched for a house in the country as a second home. When Willo and the kids got home, we looked at some of the properties but decided that we didn't need a second home. In 1971, we bought the house on Drumaldry in Bethesda, Maryland, instead. From this house, restless and uncomfortable, I left in 1972 to begin the separation that eventually resulted in our divorce in 1973.

The Outpatient Treatment Program

When the funding came to an end, I was not offered an opportunity to remain with the NIMH. I applied for and received a grant from the NIMH to set up an outpatient treatment program for alcoholics employed by the federal government. The grant had to be administered through a hospital or similar organization, so we chose to work with Washington Hospital Center, setting up an outpatient treatment center in an office building on K Street in downtown Washington, DC.

The clinical director for the treatment center was a strange and charismatic retired army psychiatrist who had not activated his MD status as a civilian. His long-term "intimate other" was also a therapist. Vince and Jane were family therapists, using their own flavor of family therapy, with trained licensed social workers on their team. They were close to Virginia Satir, an American author and therapist who was known at that time for her work in family reconstruction therapy and in family therapy treatment circles.

I wanted to be on the treatment team, but I didn't want to go through the training. Vince, Jane, and Virginia happily manipulated me because I provided a platform on which they could operate. They knew how to make me feel important; however, I was supposed to administer and bring in patients, not provide therapy. I must have realized at some subliminal level that I was being manipulated because the whole treatment-center scheme felt strange and uncomfortable.

This program was a textbook example of narcissistic excess and exploitation. We put together an exceptional staff, but it was as though the staff existed for the staff. We provided outpatient treatment for government-employee alcoholics, but our hearts and souls were with each other. We felt entitled to indulge in a range of emotional excesses funded by the NIMH. We exploited the NIMH, the Washington Hospital Center, and finally each other and ourselves.

We were like a raft of kids playing expensive mind games with someone else's money. I organized excessive training workshops for the staff, bringing in some famous and talented people to run them. This training opened up unresolved issues for several staff members, including me.

The staff training sessions led by Virginia Satir were confrontational and professional, and some of them included staff spouses. Virginia's family-reconstruction training would have been appropriate and effective if the participants had been couples who were voluntarily in treatment. That was not the case. The participants had been employed to staff a treatment center; confrontational personal therapy was not part of the job description. More than one staff member got divorced as a result of the program.

The treatment center milieu was also the trigger for my divorce. I felt that my marriage was a problem, and I wanted us to separate. I made it clear that it was nothing Willo had done; I just wanted to start over—yet again. I was still seeking something that would bring me the specialness for which I was destined, but that didn't make her feel any better.

When we opened the Alcoholism Treatment Center in 1972, I reported to the Washington Hospital Center CEO. After a few months, however, the Department of Psychiatry wanted the center to become part of their department. I was resistant and, I am sure, unpleasant.

I realize now that the Chairman of Psychiatry was a lonesome guy who just wanted to be my friend. I, however, had problems bonding, especially with authority figures. We never became friends. He committed suicide a few months later.

Because I wouldn't cooperate in the reorganization under the Department of Psychiatry, the hospital had to get rid of me. I could resign, or they would fire me. I refused to resign. My tenure with the Alcoholism Treatment Center was like a morality play about NPD. I hit all nine criteria while I was there.

I had an interesting reaction as a temporary GS-15 with the NIMH and a department administrator in a major hospital. These jobs were all below me. I wanted to be a therapist, not a manager, but I didn't want to do the work it required to become qualified as a therapist. Instead, I wanted to suddenly manifest as one. The Washington Hospital Center told me that, if I chose to be fired, I would never again work in hospital administration. However, I was special, I had gotten the grant from the NIMH, and I had created the program the hospital now wanted to give to the psychiatry department, so why would I ever want to be a hospital administrator anyway (NPD #1 through #9)?

When I declared bankruptcy a year later, Vince and Jane got stuck with a $10,000 credit union loan they had cosigned for me. It seemed appropriate. They were upset that I had fought with the hospital that eventually terminated their playground. Vince, Jane, and Virginia clearly understood my "specialness" and played it like a violin. I was their pawn and knew it but wouldn't admit it to myself. I did, however, blow the whole thing up and split, and I never paid

Vince and Jane the $10,000. Vince died of a heart attack several years later, and Jane and her son drowned while fishing in Chesapeake Bay very soon after Vince's death. No one knows how. Jane had been married to a German man during World War II and spent much of the war hiding out in the Black Forest with her son. She was a strange woman. There was a spooky quality to the Alcoholism Treatment Center experience that still makes me uneasy.

The End of My Marriage to Willo

In 1966, Willo and I bought our home on Aspen Street in northwest Washington, DC, and lived there until we moved to Drumaldry in Bethesda in 1971. The time on Aspen was as good for us as life could get with my NPD. We had friends in the neighborhood and elsewhere, we had a comfortable income, and we enjoyed life. We had a big, black Bouvier des Flandres named Deitrick. Willo had a Mercedes sports convertible, and I had a motorcycle. Willo and I worked well together, and she did everything she could to make our marriage work. She tried to get us to develop hobbies that we could do together. She was responsible for most of our friends. She loved to cook and throw parties, and we did a lot of entertaining.

While working for the NIMH, a guy who worked for me said, "You are always creating crises to solve."

He was right, and this truth hurt. All of the changes, the moves, the firings, and the starting overs were the result of my creating crises.

In 1972, Willo and I separated. Our separation had been under discussion for several months. When I told Willo in the spring that I wanted to separate, she asked me to wait until after our planned trip to Hawaii. Life went on pretty much as usual, and we made the trip. Willo did not want to end the marriage, but there was no overt anger or hostility. It was a prime example of my lack of empathy and my continual search for something better.

Willo and I negotiated a separation agreement with our attorney. We had about $10,000 in unsecured debts, and we agreed to split them and any assets. I signed the agreement but Willo did not. She had to have it notarized in Maryland, and I trusted her to get it done.

I left town for the summer; however, because Willo never signed the agreement, I had to declare bankruptcy. I could have insisted that she sign the agreement before leaving for the trip across country. The fact that I didn't insist is a good example of the fantasy world in which I lived. I did not pay attention to Willo's hidden hurt and anger. I was entitled to have everything go my way because I was special (NPD #1, #5, and #7).

The Search for Answers

In 1965, relocation back to Washington, DC, allowed me to strengthen the two strands of my quest for some sense in my life: Zen and therapy. I found a Zen group and developed a regular meditation schedule, sitting on a cushion for 20 minutes every morning. I became a disciple of Yasutani Roshi and attended several Zen meditation retreats, one of which lasted seven days and all of which were totally silent. However, as hard as I tried, I was not "getting it" with Zen.

I worked with a therapist, Sheldon Kopp, in both group and individual therapy for several years. Shelly was writing *If You Meet the Buddha on the Road, Kill Him!*[15] while I was in therapy with him. He asked Willo to write one of the chapters and she did, using her own name.

When I had to leave the group for two weeks because of a business trip to Alaska, Shelly said that, if I left for any reason, I could not return to therapy with him. I left anyway, and he threw me out. Shelly didn't want me as a patient because I was always and totally in my head with no feelings or empathy. Although NPD was not yet in the DSM, he knew that the disorder I had was not treatable. When I returned from Alaska, he referred me to Fred Klein, who had been one of his supervisees and was an excellent therapist.

Fred Klein triggered one of my first breakthroughs. I saw him on a weekly basis both individually and in a group. He asked me to lead one of our group

---

[15] Sheldon Kopp, *If You Meet the Buddha on the Road, Kill Him!* (London: Lowe & Brydon Ltd., 1974).

sessions in a chant, and about eight of us sang, "Jai Ram, Shree Ram, Jai Jai Ram." After a few minutes, I started to cry. The tears flowed and flowed, and I wept for the rest of the session. This opened up something in me that had been blocked. I have found it very easy to cry ever since, frequently tearing up with the slightest provocation. My NPD did not appear to dissipate significantly—it had no impact on my empathy block, for example—but this was clearly the beginning of a significant experience.

The end of the marriage caused a great deal of turmoil for Willo and our children Alexandra and Geoffrey. In 1982, Alex came to live with my second wife Christina and me in Santa Fe for her senior year in high school, and I have maintained a close and beautiful relationship with Alex, her husband Tom, and their boys Kyle and Ethan.

Since Christina's death in 2016, I have spent Thanksgiving and Christmas with Alex's family in Maryland. Their family works, and it is the first truly functional family I have ever known closely. The four of them treat each other with love, understanding, and respect.

The divorce put Geoff in a difficult place, and my disorder did not help. I started the separation on his sixth birthday. All the time he was growing up, I was the bad guy. Willo and I frequently argued over the child support I never fully paid. Geoff was passive-aggressive towards me; at his request, we have had several no-communication periods, each lasting for several years. I recently spent time with Geoff's four children (Julian, Liam, Max, and Sophia), two of whom I had met several times when they were very young and two of whom I had never met until recently. I am sorry that I didn't handle the divorce better, but such things are a bad show under the best of circumstances, and my disorder clearly made it worse. The lack of a relationship with my grandchildren was the result of my unwillingness to force an encounter with them against Geoff's desire as well as my inability to travel freely due to Christina's illnesses. My continuing NPD caused me to avoid difficult confrontations. I hope this has changed, and I look forward to more frequent visits to California.

I am happy to know that Geoff is a good father, with healthy affection, respect, and communication between him and his four children. I am also pleased that the cycle of weak and ineffective fathering, going back at least to my grandfather, has been broken. Geoff is showing his three sons how to be a good father under difficult circumstances, and his daughter thinks that he hung the moon. The parenting of Alex's and Geoff's families are very different, but both work. All six children are finding out who they are with no signs of NPD. Fortunately, there is no NPD gene, as far as we know now, that can be inherited, and the family genesis of the disorder is apparently not inevitable.

Christina

I met Christina Sevier, who became my second wife, when she came to work at the Alcoholism Treatment Center in Washington, DC, early in 1973. I knew from the beginning that she was exceptional, and she and I became a couple and moved in together soon after. Both of us were separated from our spouses but not yet divorced. Beautiful, highly intelligent, deeply creative, and intuitive, Christina made friends easily and was much liked by other treatment center staff. She was particularly close to one good male therapist. He and several others tried to convince her not to get into a relationship with me because they could see my NPD, even though the inclusion in the DSM was still years away. Fortunately for me, they were unsuccessful; however, I'm not sure it was fortunate for her.

I got fired, and she resigned. Christina stayed with me. We rounded up our four kids (mine plus Christina's) and a friend of Joseph's (one of Christina's children) and headed across the country in my Ford van, which, along with several tents, was our home. Of Christina's two children, Joseph was 14 years old in 1973, and Nicole was 10. Alex and Geoff were eight and six, respectively. We headed north from Washington, DC, and drove to Adams Center, New York, south of Watertown, and saw the house where my father grew up. We went north to Canada, drove west across the continent, and reentered the United States via Washington State. We then drove south down Highway 1, along the coast to Seal Beach, California, where my parents lived. We put Joseph, Nicole, and Joseph's friend on a plane back to DC and left Alex and Geoff with my parents.

Christina and I headed to Mexico. We drove down the Baja California Peninsula, through Ensenada to a beach on the Pacific side. We pitched our tent and set up camp. It was a beautiful site with big rocks, sand dunes, and coves.

There were delicious-looking mussels on the rocks, but it was the middle of the summer. We decided to observe the behavior of the Mexicans who were harvesting them. If we recognized the same people returning two days in a row, we would assume that the algae had not poisoned the mussels. We never recognized any returning mussel eaters, so we didn't harvest any. It was a wonderful place to hang out and do nothing. We had stayed in a campground near Ensenada on the way down. It was filled with pot-smoking hippies, but there were no Americans where we were. We heard that the Mexican police had plainclothes officers walking around the regular campgrounds at night, arresting pot smokers; however, there was no problem with that issue where we were camping.

After about a week, we decided to drive up to the border to make some phone calls. When we got to the inspection station on the American side, a Border Patrol officer came aboard our van to check us out. He looked in our icebox and saw that we had several mangos. When he told us that we couldn't bring fruit into the United States, we turned around, parked on the Mexican side, and walked across the border. When we walked back to the border, we saw that the Americans were using dogs to check incoming cars for drugs. We didn't pay any attention to the dogs or the officers and returned to our van on the Mexican side. When I got into the van, I noticed that the felt bag in which we kept our pot was lying in plain sight on the passenger bench. It was full of pot that we had been given by Americans who were going to cross the border and go home. Had the Border Patrol officer seen that bag, we might still be doing time in a Mexican prison.

We rented a house in Chevy Chase, Maryland, where I worked as a consultant with various organizations. Christina and I finalized our divorces. In 1975, we relocated to the Florida Keys and bought a boat with money from Christina's divorce and a loan from a friend of mine. I was not a particularly good sailor, and the boat was better for living in than for sailing. We moored it at Boot Key Marina in Marathon. I found employment as director of the

Alcoholism Treatment Center there. I also ran a weekly counseling group for adolescents. Things went well at the treatment center. I did some firing and hiring and ended up with a good staff. My counseling activities got me into trouble, however. Marathon was a conservative community of fisherman and boat people. My language and aggressive social liberalism did not go over well with the parents of my group members. I was told by the director of the center that if I didn't leave, my boat, which was dry-docked for repair, was likely to be damaged. I resigned, and Christina and I sailed our boat to Fort Lauderdale and sold it (NPD #7 and #9).

Christina and I were not yet married, but I acted as though what was hers was also mine. I used the money from the boat to start a business that didn't work. Christina was unhappy and having trouble with binge alcoholism. She left Fort Lauderdale and went to a training commune in Berkeley, California. A few months later, I collapsed my failing business and joined her for a 30-day training session. I had formed a nonprofit company to accept boats as tax-deductible contributions, which we would then fix up and sell. I also owned the van we had used to go across the country. Christina's money from the sale of our boat was now gone. I owed money to our three employees, so I left them with the company, the contributed boat, and my van. Then I took a Greyhound bus to California (NPD #6, #7, and #9).

The training center in Berkeley and the next center in Kentucky were based on the book *Handbook to Higher Consciousness*[16] by Ken Keyes, Jr. The book and the training centers were developed for the purpose of training people how to live happily by dropping or overcoming the blocks to happiness. When I scan through the book today, I see that it is filled with good observations about people and good ideas and techniques to make our lives happy. I didn't get it then, and today I know why. All that it teaches is negated by NPD. Of course, I wasn't liked or accepted in Berkeley or later in Kentucky where we lived in the commune for a year. The people with whom I was associated knew nothing about NPD, but they knew that there was something unpleasantly strange about me.

---

[16] Ken Keyes, Jr., *Handbook to Higher Consciousness,* Fifth Edition (Berkeley, CA: Living Love Center, 1975).

In 1977, at the end of the training month in Berkeley, Christina and I were married in a service at the center, which was attended by all the residents and students and officiated by Ken Keyes, Jr. The center was then dismantled, and a number of us relocated to the new center—Cornucopia—on a large tract of land in St. Mary, Kentucky. Christina was extremely popular and ran the food services for the center. I was tolerated because of her but never admitted into the "permanent resident group."

Cornucopia was a commune created to train residents how to teach Keyes's *Handbook to Higher Consciousness*. Teaching workshops were offered at the commune in Kentucky, and a school bus was modified as an RV to transport trainers throughout the country. Keyes's concepts were basically Buddhist and threefold: (1) suffering is caused by desires; (2) desires are caused by attachments (Keyes called them "addictions"); and (3) dropping the attachments rids you of the suffering.

Training involved learning what attachments are and how to drop them, including teaching the teachers how to give up their attachments. A number of processes and group activities was designed to accomplish this. The training was excellent, and much was learned about attachments. However, there was one big problem: The training didn't work for most people with deep attachments because the whole approach was intellectual and not based on an understanding of the illusion of self and how to confront that reality.

There was no meditation and no teachings regarding self-illusion and the ultimate emptiness of reality. The program failed after a couple of years because the leadership moved on to other paths. Although based on Buddhism, the failure to fully address the teachings of Buddhism was, in my opinion, the fatal flaw.

Christina and I and a close friend named Susy, who had been with us since Berkeley, decided to leave. We moved to Fort Lauderdale and rented a condominium on Ocean Boulevard. I found a job as the director of a residential drug-treatment facility. Susy and I continued to do training workshops on our own, using the techniques we had learned in Kentucky.

Bhagwan Shree Rajneesh

At the end of our stay in Kentucky in 1978, a number of us heard about a teacher in India named Bhagwan Shree Rajneesh (now Osho). I was continually searching for a solution to my discomfort and unknown disorder. I hoped that, if I became a follower of Rajneesh, he might show me the way. I was still very much in the mindset that the answers to my unrest lay elsewhere.

While in Fort Lauderdale, I sent a letter to his organization and asked to become a sannyasin.[17] They replied with my new name (Swami Anand Subodh) and included a 108-bead mala[18] with an open locket containing a picture of Rajneesh. I changed my wardrobe to all orange clothes and wore the mala until I learned what was happening at the Rajneesh Ashram in Oregon.[19] In 1982, after four years of being a sannyasin and when we were living in Santa Fe, I returned the mala and resigned from the organization. Christina had also become a sannyasin and she did the same.

Bhagwan was an interesting character. His many lectures on all known religions were brilliant and published in a collection that would fill yards of bookshelves. He grew up a Jain[20] in India but seemed to have a personal preference for Buddhism. I liked his open, no-holds-barred approach and felt that he would be a good teacher for me; however, several factors precluded my having a good experience as a follower.

Bhagwan was flawed and unable to lead the strong following that developed around him. He was terrible at picking leaders for his organization. Ma Anand Sheela, whom he chose to run the Oregon organization, was a psychopath and became the first American terrorist tried for multiple attempted murders and bioterrorism, eventually going to federal prison. Bhagwan's need to be

---

[17] A "sannyasin" is a formal disciple of Bhagwan Shree Rajneesh (Osho) who wears orange clothes and a mala; traditionally refers to a Hindu religious beggar.

[18] A "mala" is a wooden necklace, similar to a rosary, commonly used in Buddhism and Hinduism.

[19] The details of the events in the Rajneesh Ashram in Oregon are creatively examined in the movie, *Wild Wild Country*.

[20] "Jain" is a religion in India.

both cloistered and flamboyant was a major impediment to his effectiveness. The depth of his awareness and his ability to function as a religious leader are clearly open to question. After all his troubles, he changed his name to Osho. Even after his death, he still has a large and growing following, and his books continue to be printed and sold.

My expectations were a major obstacle in my discipleship about Bhagwan as my guru. Seeking a guru is dangerous because the only guru who is helpful and not hurtful is one who guides you to find the "answer" on your own. A guru can't do it for you or give you anything. I was looking for a magic solution, and there is none. Other problems were the new name, the wooden necklace, and the orange clothes. Such outward manifestations frequently get in the way of a true understanding and an epiphany, which happened to me. Bhagwan had a large following of wealthy people, European nobility, and educated members of the upper and middle class from all over the world. Had his enlightenment been deeper, he might have had an even larger and more positive impact.

No one, however, could have helped me in my spiritual quest until I understood and confronted my NPD.

In 1980, Christina and I decided to leave Fort Lauderdale and join a new center in Taos, New Mexico. This was the time of the "Earth changes" movement. Some people who had come out of the hippie-commune mentality were convinced that Earth was going to relocate on its axis, and strong winds and high water would change the face of the planet. The location of the center in Taos would supposedly survive the winds and the rising ocean, which would come inland for hundreds of miles. Christina didn't believe that the changes were coming, nor did I, but the Taos center seemed like a good idea for other reasons. I quit my job as director of a residential drug treatment program in Fort Lauderdale. We said goodbye to Susy and set off for New Mexico.

Taos and Santa Fe, New Mexico

The center was on a beautiful piece of land in the mountains above Taos. It consisted of several acres of land, a main building, and several outbuildings.

The owners were a chiropractor and his wife from Georgia. A number of people had already moved in when we arrived. I got along very well with the owner, but his wife decided that I was a threat and insisted that I leave. I'm not sure what triggered her dislike, but it was probably some manifestation of NPD.

Christina stayed in Taos while I went to Santa Fe to find us a new place to live. Santa Fe was beautiful, and I was in love with the place from day one. It would have been a wonderful final destination for Christina and me except that I screwed it all up.

I found a great house that we rented as a commune. Some of the group from Taos and the Kentucky commune joined us there. Christina and I got tired of communal living after a few months and moved into a rented apartment in town. When the commune collapsed, Christina and I bought the house and property from the original owners, who financed our purchase.

I got a job with the State of New Mexico, running the regional methadone maintenance program. Christina started her own yarn-dyeing business, using one of the outbuildings on our property. Alex came to live with us and completed her senior year in high school in Los Alamos, just up the mountain from us. Christina created a beautiful garden, and we had lots of animals: two old English sheep dogs, three horses, chickens, turkeys, geese, sheep, and rabbits. Christina hired a competent assistant, and her business thrived.

I was appreciated by the state and could have run the methadone program forever. I had a secure job with a loyal and highly competent staff. I had plenty of spare time on the job and was doing couples and individual counseling in my office with clients who were unrelated to the methadone-treatment activities.

Respected in the community, I had to actively reject attempts to put me in the guru role. Personally, I felt insecure and unfulfilled. I certainly did not feel like a guru, but I was comfortable doing counseling. I was a sannyasin of Rajneesh, so I still sported the orange clothes and mala. I had also legally changed my name to Swami Anand Subodh, the name given to me by Rajneesh. I was playing the role of being special, which made me uncomfortable.

I really wanted to develop and run a residential treatment program for alcoholics. After some thought but no discussion with Christina, I quit my job and pursued the development of a residential treatment center. In both our commune living and my desire to open a treatment center, I was trying to create a new family; however, I was not conscious of this obsession at the time.

As I mentioned, the original owners of our house had financed it for us. We could have bought them out and owned it for a $100,000 mortgage. Had I been willing to keep my job and let Christina grow her business, we could have bought up properties in Santa Fe and become multimillionaires. Christina knew this, but I was discontented; my NPD was always in the way.

I had heard that John Ehrlichman, of Watergate fame, had relocated to Santa Fe. I found his address and got his housekeeper to give me his telephone number. We got together for breakfast, and he agreed to help me develop a treatment center. John had a friend who owned a large house on several acres outside of Santa Fe, which he was willing to vacate for our center. We were moving along nicely. We even had a physician, an Alcoholics Anonymous (AA) member, who agreed to be the medical director.

The owner of the property, who was going to underwrite much of the project, had a friend—his confessor, a Catholic priest, and an AA member. At this time, I was giving up being a disciple of Rajneesh and putting away my orange clothes. The priest interviewed me and was satisfied that I was through with Rajneesh and didn't have any leftover poisonous beliefs. One day, however, the priest saw me in an orange T-shirt under my jacket. The scandals from the Rajneesh Ashram in Oregon were all over the news, and he was convinced that I was a dangerous undercover Rajneeshee.[21] The priest told his friend not to have anything more to do with me. John's friend offered me $25,000 to give up my interest in the project and go away. I needed the money, but I was determined to build a treatment center, so I turned him down and proceeded without him.

John Ehrlichman and I spent a lot of time together while we were developing the project. We discussed his experience at the White House and in prison and the books he had just written. During our relationship, it was interesting

---

[21] A "Rajneeshee" is a follower of Bhagwan Shree Rajneesh (Osho).

that I could never forget myself and just get to know John. He was open and willing to discuss anything; I was self-absorbed and self-concerned, never allowing myself to get close to John or to fully appreciate the interesting life he had lived. With most people, it was like my sister had said: I couldn't see beyond my own nose. It was certainly that way with John (NPD #1, #2, and #7).

In 1982, I proceeded with my compulsion to create a treatment center, which I would call Amethyst Hall. I raised enough money to get the project started by selling stock to a number of well-connected people in Santa Fe. I found a large ranch north of Santa Fe on the Rio Grande that was already set up to be a retreat center and could become a residential treatment center with minor renovations.

As I was entering the Bank of Santa Fe to apply for a loan, I met the president of the bank.

"I need $50,000," I said to him as he was coming out of the door.

He turned, and I followed him into the bank to a desk in the lobby.

"Get Larry $50,000!" he told the woman at the desk.

That's all there was to it. I hired a good staff, furnished the place with taste and style, and opened the doors of Amethyst Hall. We chose the name because the amethyst stone is a mythological cure for alcoholism. Amethyst Hall turned out to be a mythological cure also.

It should have been a success. If I had done the marketing right or had hired someone else to do it, and if I had been a good administrator, we would have done well; however, in reality, I was not at all ready to be successful. I was frightened about what I had gotten myself into, and I was manifesting all the NPD characteristics at once. I was in a great deal of physical and mental anguish. I ran the place into the ground by not developing a viable marketing program and by not providing competent leadership as the CEO. Both of these deficiencies could have been addressed had I been able to recognize them and bring in competent people to assist me. My board of directors finally fired me. They couldn't turn the business around, so they sold the property, and it became an extension of a hospital in town (NPD #1, #2, #7, and #9).

My NPD was in full-flowing manifestation in Santa Fe, often coming out in humorous ways. Christina's son Joseph lived in Santa Fe with his wife-to-be Livia Page-Phillips. They had met in Oregon at the Rajneesh Ashram, which had become so controversial. They got married at our house with the service in our living room. Livia's mother and uncle came from England. I was into watching major movies on cassette every night. I thought that showing a movie to all the wedding guests would be a fine idea. So, after the wedding service, I set up the television and played *Patton*. Everyone seemed to enjoy it, but I got ribbed for years for showing an anti-English movie to Livia's family and for dominating the postwedding festivities. If anyone noticed that Patton and I seemed to have the same disorder, they didn't mention it (NPD #7).

Christina was trying to run her company and support the family since my income was minimal to nonexistent. She finally had to close her business because she could not use her income to expand and compete.

I was hired as the administrator for a small company that had bought a nursing-home building and created a psychiatric hospital near downtown Santa Fe. I got the building renovated, the staff hired, and the hospital operating. All went well at first until the original owner sold it to a company that owned a number of hospitals. After seeing me at work for several months and observing my supervisory style with staff and my attitude toward physicians, the new company's regional director decided that I needed to go. I'm sure that I was simply too self-absorbed to do what was most effective and profitable for the company. At the time, I was outraged; however, when I look back, I realize that they were justified in getting rid of me.

Out of work again, I was able to find employment as a car salesman in Santa Fe. This led to an assistant sales manager job in Houston, which I gave up when I was offered a position as Director of Finance and Insurance at a car dealership in Santa Fe. Christina remained at our Santa Fe home during my brief employment in Houston. I had three director jobs with auto dealerships—two in Santa Fe and one in Albuquerque. I didn't fit in well with the car company crowd, and I wasn't well liked. I was good at what I did in the finance department, but my bosses and peers felt that I was not one of them. I was always eventually fired. Again, it was the NPD that got me in trouble. I don't really know what manifestations of NPD kept getting me fired, but lack of empathy and a focus only on myself were probably at the heart of people's dislike of having me around.

In 1990, when I had used up all the job opportunities available, we sold our home in Santa Fe and rented an apartment in Albuquerque. I was fired in Albuquerque because the manager wanted to hire a friend to take my job. That was the stated reason; I now realize that it was the NPD again. I had spent the last decades thinking that I was searching for something outside of myself; in actuality, I was fleeing from something inside me.

We began the new decade by driving to Melbourne, Florida, where someone I'd known in the alcoholism-treatment business offered me a job. We rented an attractive apartment on the bank of the Intracoastal Waterway. The new company was contracting with alcoholism-treatment programs to take over their admissions function and increase their census. I was responsible for finding new business by phone. I had met Billy, the manager, in California when he was running a navy treatment program. He was a bright, creative guy but clearly a sociopath. He had been running a treatment hospital in Melbourne for several years that was owned by a large corporation. His sociopathy had caught up with him, and he had been let go.

Billy was a habitual liar, which probably did him in. He started this new company and hired me to do the marketing. I was quite successful, and we were doing well for a while. Eventually, his personality became a problem with some of our client hospitals. Billy was always good to me, but he was deceptive and manipulative as well as controlling. I was never able to relate effectively to authority figures, but I wanted to destroy Billy. He may well have reminded me of my own disorders. For whatever psychological reasons, I set out to replace him in a very naïve and flawed manner.

One of our clients was a hospital in Miami. I set up a meeting with the CEO, and we met in her office. Sensing that something was not quite right, she intuitively asked one of her staff to join us. I laid out my proposal: Since Billy was flawed, I would take over the hospital's contract and run it myself. The CEO was taken aback. She asked me to leave and had me escorted out of the hospital. She called Billy, and I resigned. This incident is a blatant example of my NPD (NPD #1, #2, #5, and #7).

Undaunted, I set up my own company to do the same thing. This was successful until one of my senior colleagues got fed up with me, arranged a meeting with our funding source, and got me fired. I now realize that he just got fed up with my NPD behavior.

My last job in Florida was as Director of Business Development at the University Behavioral Center in Orlando. I commuted to this job from Melbourne. The job lasted about a year. It was the same old story. I failed to bond with the hospital administrator. I was more concerned with myself than I was with making sure that my department responded to the needs of the hospital and the directions of the administrator. I was offered a job in Louisiana at the same time that the administrator was ready to fire me. We parted friends.

I Discover Narcissistic Personality Disorder

Christina had been seeing a therapist in Melbourne whom she liked very much. She had been in counseling with a psychiatrist when I met her, but that was never successfully concluded. She had a number of unresolved issues stemming from her difficult original family milieu. She asked me to have a session alone with her therapist. This kind of request was not unusual, so I went to see her and gave it little thought.

Shortly thereafter, Christina and I had an unusual discussion. We were in our apartment in Melbourne one evening in 1993. Christina had told her therapist that she thought I had NPD. After meeting with me, her therapist confirmed her suspicion. She advised Christina not to confront me, however, because she said that I would deny the diagnosis and nothing positive would come from the confrontation. The therapist explained that it was not possible to treat a person with NPD because they would never recognize that there was anything wrong with them. Fortunately for me, Christina did not take her recommendation.

I was watching television in our apartment when Christina handed me some pages to read, including the section in the DSM on NPD. As I read the description of the disorder, I broke out in a cold sweat. It was a mirror. *It was me.* Flashback tableaus appeared—classic examples of NPD. I never doubted the diagnosis then or since.

Suddenly, my crazy and confused life of serial failures and stupid actions made sense. I was able to accept the fact of my NPD because my life had been such a consistent series of failures. Had I been prosperous and successful, which many people with NPD are, there would have been no reason for me to question my behavior. I would have rejected the diagnosis even if people who knew me well could see clearly that I fit the criteria. The world is full of people with NPD who are incapable of changing because they can't see a problem. I could accept that I was manifesting the nine characteristics, however, because I remembered time after time when one of those characteristics had brought me to ruin.

Christina revealed the secret that was not a secret to anyone who had known me: My disorder had a name and a list of distinguishing characteristics.

I also had a "muscle memory" of playing the NPD game all my life. Recognizing that I had NPD was one thing; dropping the strong attachment to my dysfunctional self was another.

I had been attempting to practice Zen Buddhism for decades. I had a good intellectual understanding of the history and philosophy of Zen. It was now very clear that NPD and the practice of Zen Buddhism were diametrically opposed due to the dysfunctional illusion of a separate and permanent self or ego.

The core of the disorder for a person with NPD is summed up in this statement: "I am a self, separate from other selves, which is permanent, special, unique, and worthy of admiration." The person with NPD views their reality through the prism of this illusion. Because of the disorder, they will never question the permanent reality of the illusion. The task of disidentifying from the "illusory separate self" is at the heart of many spiritual paths, and the "normal" human being can at least question if the self is an illusion.

For the person with NPD, however, being arrogant, haughty, and ultimately lacking in empathy are experienced as part of the human condition and not a manifestation caused by a disorder. The person with NPD does not consciously experience any of the nine characteristics. I knew there was something wrong with me, but I was never aware of manifesting a disorder.

When I accepted my NPD, I accepted the fact that giving up the illusion of a separate and permanent self was necessary, but I didn't know how to do it. I also didn't know how to find out how to do it. I clearly understood from my intellectual study that the development of an ego is necessary for normal growth. Also, the illusion of a "self" ("I" or "me") that is "ours" is common, and important, for adolescents.

However, the reality is that we are heart/mind. The human aggregates that are labeled as "self" are just feelings. When adults identify the self aggregates as something separate or special, they are creating the feeling of suffering that the Buddha taught was unnecessary. The person with NPD has a disorder of the feelings that cannot be self-conscious. Having lived for 58 years with this illusion, how was I to drop it? Intellectual understanding was apparently not the path to that change of perception.

Alexandria and Monroe, Louisiana

In 1994, when my job in Orlando was concluding, I was offered a job in Alexandria, Louisiana, as the CEO of a psychiatric hospital. I moved to Alexandria while Christina stayed in Melbourne for another six months. The CEO job lasted a year, and I was finally fired for all the same reasons as the earlier terminations. I didn't bond or communicate well with my boss, and I was not trained to be a CEO.

After seven months of unemployment, I was hired as the CEO of a psychiatric hospital in Monroe, Louisiana. Christina stayed in our house in Alexandria, and I lived in a travel trailer in Monroe, driving the hundred miles home every weekend. The Monroe hospital job was more successful; however, after a year, the hospital was sold and the new owner fired me. He then tried to replace me with two of my staff and finally closed the hospital.

We have a wonderful house in Alexandria, with an amazing garden that Christina created. I didn't want to move. I came home and started my own company. Since 1997, I have had a recruiting company, and we find candidates to fill jobs in behavioral healthcare. I am still running Larry White Associates, Inc. I have several staff members and no longer have to produce all the revenue by myself. The nearly two decades (from 1997 until Christina's death in 2016) were good ones for me, but not so much for Christina. Christina's creativity in designing the garden and decorating and furnishing the house were wonderful. Most of all, Christina was a multitude who deepened my life and brought me beauty, peace, and understanding. I miss her very much.

Our experience in Alexandria was very different for Christina. While we were apart for six months, Christina had blossomed in Melbourne. She continued to see her therapist, who she thought was helpful to her. She worked out regularly in a gym and joined a yoga group. She joined a dance group and made some friends with whom she socialized regularly. She cleaned up her diet, lost weight, and quit drinking. When it was time for her to come to Alexandria and help me pick out a house for us, she was resistant to moving. It was not possible for me to maintain two residences on my salary, and I didn't know where I could find work in Florida. I was enthusiastic about the Alexandria opportunity and looked forward to becoming a part of the community. Christina's therapist told her that, if she didn't leave me, our relationship would kill her, but I didn't think we had any alternatives except to move to Alexandria.

Christina said we would die in Alexandria. She said it was easy to get stuck in a place like this, and we would never be able to leave. She didn't like small southern towns, and she had a hard time finding friends with whom she could bond. However, we were here to stay. She joined the garden club and became its president. Christina poured her creativity into the garden, the house, her embroidery, and basketry. She continued to be a voracious reader.

After a few years, she began to eat compulsively and put on a lot of weight, which led to a series of health problems and operations. We bought a series of campers and, in spite of Christina's increasing illnesses, we went RV camping in Texas and Arkansas. We made 13 trips to South Padre Island alone.

During the last few years of her life, Christina spent most of the time in her big recliner in the television room. She developed diabetes and liver disease. She had back trouble, which led to an operation. She had triple bypass surgery because of heart problems. New issues kept emerging, and old problems got worse and worse. There seemed to be no solutions. She died on December 13, 2016, of heart-related problems.

Christina was a wonderful wife and a wonderful friend and companion. Our marriage changed my life and saved my life by helping me confront my NPD. Against the advice of close friends, her brother, and her therapist, Christina married me and stayed with me. There is no doubt that my NPD had a profound and negative effect upon her life. I will always be deeply grateful for her love and loyalty. Christina rescued me from NPD.

The backyard had begun as a green lawn with one lonely tree. Thanks to Christina, now there is an office/apartment and a wonderfully designed garden. The 60-foot willow tree is the result of a three-foot branch that Christina planted after using it in a presentation that won Best in Show at the annual Alexandria Garden Club exhibit in 1994.

My life with Christiana in Alexandria was an important time for my journey out of NPD. I have mentioned my lifelong history of anger and rage, which manifested from time to time but always existed beneath the surface of my personality. When I worked in the garden and got hot, sweaty, and tired, the rage would boil up inside. I never blew up or mentioned it, but it was there. The rage had nothing to do with Christina and was a typically latent but permanent part of my disorder.

One day, right before I flew to California for one of my biannual trips to visit my mother, I felt that some change had taken place.

I thought, "I have nothing to offer my family in California, and I don't want anything from them."

The reception I got in California was new. My mother, sister, and brother-in-law had always been painfully aware of my anger. Now they felt different, and they wanted to spend time with me while I was there. The anger and rage were gone. When I returned to Alexandria, I never again felt rage when I was working in the garden or anger at any time. The anger and rage had simply dropped out of my life.

What happened to all the anger and rage? Where did it come from in the first place? This is a good question and one with which I have struggled. The anger and rage were always free floating and never consistently specific. The anger was always there. It would manifest specifically from time to time, and then retreat into a kind of background radiation.

Other people could often see or feel this background radiation, but I was seldom aware of it or I was aware of it like a constant pain to which I learned not to pay attention. I think the anger was the result of my becoming aware of the disorder that was finally identified as NPD.

I am not sure when I first became aware of this problem and created the anger and rage, but I think it happened at Deep Springs after I had left home for the first time. The anger and rage influenced my activities in conscious and unconscious ways. I realize that I avoided buying guns until after I was consciously aware of NPD because I was afraid of what I might do with them to other people. I was aware of "road rage," which would emerge from time to time.

When I finally dropped the anger and rage on that day in our garden before I flew to California, it was gone. Since that day, I have not experienced or manifested any anger or rage regardless of the circumstances. The most frequent opportunities to observe this lack of anger are on the road. When some driver does a stupid thing that would have stimulated anger or rage previously, I just shrug or smile. I don't have to consciously suppress anger; it just isn't there anymore.

As I mentioned, three experiences freed me from the shackles of NPD: (1) in a group therapy session, I opened myself up to being able to cry; (2) Christina got me in touch with my NPD; and (3) I dropped the rage. The fourth and final event in my journey through NPD was a Zen experience, the result of which allowed me to drop my inability to understand empathy.

Zen in the End

Starting a Zen Group in Monroe

Soon after I took the CEO job at the psychiatric hospital in Monroe in 1996, I interviewed a psychiatrist for the staff named Rusty Ragsdill. He turned out to be a Zen Buddhist, so I hired him. We decided to start a Zen group. We set up a meeting by advertising in a local Monroe bookstore and got a decent number of people to come and check us out.

When the dust settled, we had two people as regular sitters in addition to Rusty and me. Gary and Ann Findley were both local college professors. They had been participating for several years in an annual Rinzai Zen retreat led by the Japanese Rinzai Roshi Keido Fukushima. The retreat was held at a beautiful center in Arkansas. We set up a weekly Zen sit on Thursdays, followed by coffee and discussion at Books-A-Million in Monroe. None of us wanted to discuss Zen explicitly, and Fukushima Roshi didn't want us to discuss Zen, so we stuck to national politics.

In 1997, because of my experience with Zen study and practice, Fukushima Roshi accepted me as a koan student. This was the first retreat where he had accepted any koan students. He required that students attend three of his retreats before entering koan study. He allowed me to start koan study at my first retreat because of my previous experience with Yasutani Roshi. I attended five retreats in six years before he discontinued his visits to the United States. He started me through the Mu koan. Koan study is a long process. There are over 100 checking koans in Mu. This study with a Master proceeds for years until the understanding of the student has been passed by the Master for the full array of koans in the tradition of the Master.

Fukushima Roshi used the same process with his disciples on the Arkansas retreats as he used with his monastic and lay disciples in Kyoto at his monastery Tōfuku-ji. The experiences with Fukushima Roshi were significant and important, and I am sorry that they had to end. He died of Parkinson's disease in March 2011 at the age of 78. Fukushima Roshi was an internationally known calligrapher, and I am privileged to have one of his "Mu" calligraphies, which I watched him create. It was a rare opportunity to know and work with Fukushima Roshi.

When I dropped out of the Monroe group in 2008, I was living in Alexandria and driving to Monroe once a week. I was anxious to start a zazenkai[22] in Alexandria. Richard Collins, a newly appointed dean at Louisiana State University in Alexandria, was to give a lecture on Zen cartoons at the museum in Alexandria. When about 12 people and I showed up at the museum, we discovered that the lecture was cancelled due to the threat of a tropical storm. I insisted that we call Richard and get him to talk to us anyway. He came with some bottles of wine, and we moved into the nearby offices of an architect who had come to the lecture. We had a good discussion, and Richard delivered the full lecture a few weeks later at the museum.

Richard had been a student of Robert Livingston, who was the abbot of the New Orleans Zen Temple,[23] until just before Katrina. I pushed hard for the Alexandria group and encouraged Richard to make it happen. Although I had accepted the reality of my NPD in 1994, I was still very much in its thrall.

I was outspoken in the group and wanted to be its de facto leader. I thought that I was intellectually well grounded in Zen. I had a long history of Zen meditation and discipleship with two Japanese Roshis. I knew theoretically that the illusion of a separate self was a barrier to enlightenment, and I knew that I was attached to my illusory self. I didn't realize the depth of my attachment or how significantly my NPD distorted my experience with Zen.

---

[22] A "zazenkai" (also called a "sangha") is a Zen meditation group.

[23] The New Orleans Zen Temple is a Soto temple in the lineage of Kōdō Sawaki and Taisen Deshimaru.

In spite of my ignorance, or probably because of it, I lectured and brow-beat the Zen group about the meaning and practice of Zen at every available opportunity.

In spite of my attitude and behavior, we had a strong group of about 10 and sometimes as many as 15 people, who were all committed to weekly sitting meditation, if not to Zen. Richard was a good and gentle leader, and he did not "push" Zen. He was, however, very available to discuss Zen for those who wanted to learn about it.

In 2010, two of my fellow group members, Margaret and Bob, asked Richard to arrange for their lay ordination at the New Orleans Zen Temple. I had resisted the idea of ordination since it had never been a part of the Zen practice to which I was accustomed. I didn't want to oppose it, so I joined the group to be ordained as a bodhisattva.[24]

This is from the ordination ceremony: "The bodhisattva ordination cer-emony does not mark a destination reached. On the contrary, this is only one turn in this garden of forking paths, our life; a pause that points to a continuing dedication to the way of the bodhisattva: to help all beings by serving the sang-ha,[25] to serve the sangha by helping all beings, to serve all beings by doing zazen."

This ceremony was an important experience for the three of us, who were ordained as bodhisattvas, and for Richard, who received his ordination as a priest/monk. The ordination experience transformed the Alexandria group. The four of us wore black robes, and the New Orleans Zen Temple ceremonies became part of the meditation activities. These changes resulted in the depar-ture on the part of those meditators who were not committed to Zen.

Richard had been very helpful and much appreciated by all of us—both Zen and non-Zen meditators—but he left soon after these changes in the med-itation group and moved to the West Coast where he became Dean of Arts and Humanities at California State University, Bakersfield.

---

[24] A "bodhisattva" is a person who is able to reach nirvana (ultimate postdeath enlightenment) but delays doing so out of compassion in order to save all suffering beings.

[25] A "sangha" (also called a "zazenkai") is a Zen meditation group.

The ceremonies have a real and subtle significance, which relates to the context of the sitting environment and to the fact that they are performed at all of the sanghas in the lineage. Richard always made it clear that the significance of the ceremonies was not spiritual.

In an attempt to meet the needs of the majority of the original group of meditators, in 2013, I set up a midweek meditation at another location with no ceremony or rituals. I had left the Sunday meetings to pursue the no-ceremonies group and to get in touch with my struggle regarding the relation of NPD and Zen practice. The no-ceremonies group continues to meet on Saturday morning in the same location as the Sunday zazen of the Zen Fellowship of Alexandria.

My temporary departure from the Sunday group lasted about three years and was necessary and helpful; my return was timely and appropriate. Richard Collins has been given Dharma[26] transmission (Shiho[27]) and is now the abbot of the New Orleans Zen Temple. Bob Savage was ordained as a priest/monk and is the leader of the Zen Fellowship of Alexandria. The Sawaki/Deshimaru lineage is small but strong in America and can be expected to have a significant influence as Zen in America continues to grow and mature.

The End of Narcissistic Personality Disorder

My recovery began in 1994 when Christina confronted me with the reality of my NPD. My acceptance of this reality gave me helpful insights into my life and why it had evolved as it had. I already had a good intellectual understanding of the illusion of self and how it blocked any experience of wholeness; however, I was still impaired by NPD and confused about my experience of self.

After moving to Alexandria, I failed as a CEO in two hospitals because of my lack of empathy and my inability to face the challenges of the job or to perform effectively. I was still "special." It is also important to note that my

---

[26] "Dharma" are teachings of the Buddha.

[27] "Shiho" is a Soto Zen Master ordination. After Shiho, the title "Roshi" can be used.

feelings of inadequacy and inferiority, which I believe are endemic to NPD, contributed significantly to my failures as a CEO.

If self-consciousness is impaired, as it certainly is in NPD, then seeing through self is seemingly impossible. Being haughty or arrogant was part of my makeup that did not spontaneously go away with my understanding that I had NPD. Willo and I used to say that we didn't want to associate socially with anyone who had not been in counseling or psychotherapy. We felt that some level of self-awareness was necessary in order to have a social relationship.

There is great truth to this idea, but I used it as an arrogant sense of being more aware than most people. In writing this narrative, I realize that I have been haughty and arrogant in my relationships with people for most of my life. I always said that I didn't want to "small talk." I am known in Alexandria for wanting to discuss politics even though it is socially taboo. My demand for "substantive" conversations was a means of keeping my conversations impersonal and intellectual where I could dominate. So-called "small talk" is intimate and personal. It requires the participants to pay attention to their interlocutors rather than only on the rhetoric or the ideas. I have recently started to appreciate the dimensions of "small talk."

Last year, a friend started a weekly luncheon for several of his longtime friends. During one of our lunches, I noticed that a woman in the group was uncomfortable with political talk. For the first time in my life, I faced the fact that I had three ways to proceed: (1) I could ignore her discomforts and talk about anything I wanted to (as I always have); (2) I could drop out of the group (and avoid the issue); or (3) I could, in deference to her feelings, avoid subjects that made her feel uncomfortable (a concession I had seldom made in the past).

I chose the last option, and I am glad that I did. The lunches have been enjoyable, and I am learning to relate to people socially on a personal and caring basis. I had not realized that I had never done that on a regular basis for my whole life. Haughty arrogance was a habit. Regular zazen softens these habits. It is possible, however, that zazen in the grip of NPD actually reinforces the NPD.

The first step in the path of recovery for the NPD sufferer is to recognize the problem intellectually. This step is almost never taken. Even if it is taken, a great deal of work lies ahead before the habits of a lifetime can be dropped.

Had I not been moving to a new job and community when Christina introduced me to the reality of my NPD, I would have immediately started counseling with a psychotherapist; however, psychotherapy could only be part of the transformation. As it was, I struggled with the reality of NPD without knowing how to drop the illusion for 22 years.

My existential concern about the "self" lay beneath the surface of my awareness before I learned about my NPD, although I was intellectually aware that the self was an illusion. As time went on, I became increasingly concerned about finding a way to drop the illusion. I was outspoken about the apparent failure of Zen teachers to address the problem and to help members of their groups to confront the issue of the illusory self. Again, this was a manifestation of NPD: blaming someone else for my lack of understanding.

While I now suspect that I was wrong because of the subtlety of the Zen Master/disciple relationship, I still suspect that the illusion of self is frequently underregarded in many American Zen groups. I say that I would have started psychotherapy had I not moved, but perhaps I was fortunate. Much, if not most, psychotherapy and counseling is simply "tuning the self."

In November 2015, I had an experience that led to moving beyond the NPD into a new place of love, openness, and growth. I became immediately aware of experiences of empathy, which were new to me. How simple and how monumental! The experience was sudden, rapid, and visual. It was a vision of the illusory self disappearing. Although this is a genuine Zen experience, it is not the experience of the "selfless self" of kensho.[28]

This was an end to NPD, and my "disorder" was gone. Narcissistic personality traits remain, but they can be addressed in continued zazen. An opening now appears to be present to experience what the Buddha and all the patriarchs of Zen have taught; however, no one can be more opaque to self-awareness than the individual with NPD.

---

[28] "Kensho" (or "satori") means enlightenment.

My struggle to free myself from the illusion of self had become strong; in fact, I was quite disturbed that I could not extricate myself from it. I had been reading *Awakening to Infinite Presence: The Clarity of Self-Realization*[29] by Robert Wolfe. His book was an interesting trigger for me. From a Zen perspective, his story is superficial and, in my opinion, he doesn't "get it." He considers himself enlightened because he intellectually sees the self as an illusion and identifies with ultimate reality as he understands it. I was appalled by the shallowness of his understanding. However, his book did seem to be the final trigger that resulted in the experience I discussed above. After my experience, I turned several people on to the book in the naïve hope that it would be a trigger for them too, but it fell completely flat. Triggers are individual, special, and nonrational.

In April 2015, I had finished one of the most influential books in my history of reading Zen: *The Third Turning of the Wheel: Wisdom of the Samdhinirmocana Sutra*[30] by Reb Anderson. The reading of this book may have helped prepare me for my experience in November; however, the triggers for Zen experiences are different for everyone.

The experience that I had was one of wordless understanding. I felt great relief and, for the first time in my life, my understanding was not just intellectual. The world felt different. The first big change was the feeling of empathy, which I had never felt before.

It was close to Christmas, and the next day I took Christina to shop at a store I had never liked. I always saw the store as pompously conservative and in-your-face Christian. The store was enormous and specialized in every possible variety of hobby supply that anyone could imagine. Christina always liked to go there to get Christmas decorating supplies. She was riding in her electric scooter; I was walking behind, pushing the shopping cart. As we approached the checkout line, I suddenly realized that I didn't have my usual hate for the

---

[29] Robert Wolfe, *Awakening to Infinite Presence: The Clarity of Self-Realization* (Ojai, CA: Karina Library Press, 2015).

[30] Reb Anderson, *The Third Turning of the Wheel: Wisdom of the Samdhinirmocana Sutra* (Berkeley, CA: Rodmell Press, 2012).

place. For the first time, I saw the store as attractive and pleasant and the people as friendly and lovable. It was a new and strange feeling.

I continued to experience things differently. Instead of feeling contempt for the morbidly obese people in the mall, I felt compassion and realized that they were brave to just carry on with their lives as they were doing. I realized I had given up the dread that had been part of my life for as long as I could remember. I was experiencing empathy for the first time. I was happy and felt completed and comfortable in a new way. This feeling has grown and deepened since 2015 as I have continued my practice of zazen.

NPD is usually associated with highly successful people who are difficult to work with but who must be taken seriously because of their power and position. People in this category are almost universally not open to recognizing their disorder or accepting the need for change. However, I am sure that there are many ordinary, inconspicuous people who are struggling with NPD and have no idea what is wrong with them or what to do about their suffering. I use the word "suffering" because NPD is an unpleasant disorder for everyone who has it, regardless of their power, position, or station in life. Beneath the surface of the person with NPD is a frightened and insecure individual who is attempting to convince the world to convince him that he is "okay."

Why Zen?

Why did I become deeply attracted to Zen Buddhism while I was at Deep Springs in 1953? There must have been some unconscious intuition that kept me struggling with Zen for over 40 years. Perhaps meditating all those years between 1960 and 1994 prepared me to be open to the existence of my NPD. Zen practice allowed me to experience a vision of the illusory self disappearing that has apparently resolved my NPD. In writing this book, I have come to appreciate my NPD, which has been such a dramatic impetus for change.

The end of my NPD has afforded me the opportunity to discover Zen in a new way. It is not possible to experience NPD and understand or practice Zen with any depth or conviction. No two views of "reality" could be more diametrically opposed. Thus, my experience of Zen practice is very different and much more intense than it has ever been. If it was necessary for me to struggle with NPD in order to struggle with the meaning of "self" and find Zen, with all that has and will imply, then I am grateful for my long adventure with NPD and thankful for my opportunity to more fully experience what Zen has to teach.

It is important to mention that my ability to have fun has increased incrementally with the end of my disorder. I now live alone and enjoy doing so. I enjoy being with friends and doing things just for fun, like reading serious and nonserious books in a wide variety of subjects. In the NPD days, everything I did had to have a positive point or meaning, which is the opposite of having fun. I am increasingly enjoying just being, hanging out, and doing what feels like being done at the moment. I am doing things that have meaning for me, or are fun for me, and are not prescribed by some "model" of what should or should not be done. My relationships with people are different. I am more aware and more empathetic, and I am more able to form strong friendships. Most importantly, there is a lighter and more joyous tone about everything I do now. Since I am no longer under the shroud of NPD, I am discovering a new world of Zen practice.

Afterword by
Jeffrey Rouse, MD

When I began specialty training to become a psychiatrist, my first patients were the temporary residents of an acute psychiatric hospital. These wards and units are the net into which society casts persons at their most despondent, their most disturbed, and their most disordered.

In diagnostic assessments, I encountered strange, illogical modes of thought, whirlpools consuming mental attention at strong variance to my own understanding of the universe, systems of belief strongly suggestive of a malfunctioning brain. I was taught that these "fixed, false beliefs" are correctly termed "delusions," and my acculturation into my new specialty made this term an everyday part of my vocabulary. Delusions became, then, a possible symptom to be assessed in all patients, a binary state: delusions were either present or absent.

Later in training did I treat the outpatients, persons functioning well enough to at least not have to sleep in a hospital under 24-hour observation. In clinic settings, there was one personality disorder that I did not get to meet: narcissistic personality disorder. Persons with true NPD are like a rare endangered species in the mental health world; you know they exist because the books assert their existence, but they are rarely captured in the wild, so to speak. If I had evaluated a person with NPD, my initial evaluation would have included the statement "no delusions were elicited." I would have presented the case to my attending supervising psychiatrist, and that statement would not have been questioned. I might have been told the time-honored psychiatric trope that narcissists don't stay in treatment, and it doesn't matter because there is no "cure."

When I read Larry White's manuscript, it upended my expectations, for not only is it a rare, unflinching self-examination and life-accounting from an NPD survivor, but one that asserts a cure: not from the analyst's couch but from a zafu.[31] Also, his account seemed at variance with the patient, humorous, self-effacing author whom I had met at a sesshin.[32] At no point as we spoke did my "psychiatric alarm bells" start ringing to suggest that I was interacting with a narcissist caught in the dojo.[33] However, Larry's book makes clear that his life's struggle is, ultimately, an example writ large of the universal chafing we all experience at the boundaries of our true Delusion, the fixed, false belief that "we" exist.

—Jeffrey Rouse, MD
Assistant Professor of Forensic Psychiatry, Tulane University

---

[31] A "zafu" is a cushion used for meditation.

[32] A "sesshin" is a Zen meditation retreat.

[33] A "dojo" (also known as a "zendo") is a room where zazen is practiced.

About the Author

Larry White has been the president of his own business since 1997. Larry White Associates, Inc. is a personnel placement business that finds candidates for hospital and clinic employers. Prior to starting his own business, Larry was a psychiatric hospital administrator and a director of alcohol- and substance-abuse treatment programs. He has been a practitioner of Zen Buddhism since college and a disciple of Hakuun Yasutani Roshi and Keido Fukushima Roshi. Larry was born in California and has lived in Boston; Washington, DC; Virginia; Florida; and New Mexico. He now lives in Louisiana and continues to run his business and participate in the activities of two Zen groups.

Acknowledgements

This book "emerged" from a long telephone conversation with my friend Mickey DeKeyser. It was not something that had been long planned or anticipated; it was a project that suddenly became the right thing to do. Mickey planted the seed, which quickly grew into a major project for me. Writing this book was both painful and rewarding, and the support and suggestions I received from friends and family who read and commented on the various versions of the manuscript were much appreciated.

Special thanks go to Richard Collins without whose support and encouragement I probably would not have proceeded. His editorial assistance greatly strengthened the initial manuscript. When it became clear that the publishing community was not standing in line to publish my book, two old friends and fellow disciples of the late Fukushima Roshi—Gary Findley and Rusty Ragsdill—came back into my life and helped with additional revisions and suggestions. All of you played crucial roles in bringing this project to fruition.

Finally, I want to thank Joanne Shwed of Backspace Ink for her creativity and expertise in bringing this book to final publication. I feel very fortunate to have discovered Joanne. She is a delight to work with.

Printed in Great Britain
by Amazon

61356223R00058